Edited by E.I. Hernández-Jiménez, E.M. Rakhanskaya

I0096798

PIGMENTATION

IN COSMETIC DERMATOLOGY & SKINCARE PRACTICE

Cosmetics & Medicine
Publishing

Author/Editor:

Elena I. Hernández-Jiménez, *Ph.D.*

Editor:

Ekaterina M. Rakhanskaya, *M.D.* Neurologist, radiation safety specialist

Author:

Vera I. Albanova, *M.D., Ph.D., Prof.* Dermatologist

PIGMENTATION IN THE COSMETIC DERMATOLOGY AND SKINCARE PRACTICE

Pigment spots are the third most common issue addressed by skincare specialists. Both young and elderly clients come with this complaint, many not for the first time. Therefore, specialists who can effectively resolve these problems will undoubtedly be in demand and will achieve well-deserved recognition.

This book provides complete and reliable information that will help you build a truly effective and safe program for treating pigmented lesions. The book consists of four parts. The first part describes the nature and mechanisms of pigmentation formation, both constitutive (fixed genetically) and facultative (caused by internal or external influences). The stages of melanogenesis, the current understanding of melanocyte physiology and melanin functions, and differences in skin types between people of different ethnic groups are discussed in detail. Special attention is given to factors influencing pigmentation: hormones, stress, inflammation, nutrients, and ultraviolet radiation. Moreover, "new" factors, such as visible light, infrared radiation, and air pollutants, are discussed clearly and comprehensively. This part concludes with a chapter on the evolution of pigmentation. All this information will give you an in-depth understanding of the nature of pigmentation lesions and, thus, the possibilities of effectively combating them.

The second part presents clinical types of dyschromia and describes methods for assessing pigmentation.

The third and largest part of the book is devoted to methods of pigmentation prevention and treatment available in skincare practice. Modern depigmenting and exfoliating cosmetic products and the dermal targets on which they act are discussed in detail. Also covered are outdated and dangerous ingredients that can still be found on the market. Separate sections are devoted to sunscreens and antioxidants because they are no less important than bleaching agents in the modern concept of working with pigmentation lesions. Furthermore, in this part, the possibilities of physical methods are discussed with a detailed description of lasers and IPL devices. These methods allow both pigment-producing and pigment-distributing cells of superficial and deep lesions to be targeted. Injection procedures are also touched upon, focusing on their real possibilities and risks, as well as nutraceuticals for skin lightening with proven effectiveness.

The last, fourth part, is devoted to treating vitiligo as the most common variant of hypomelanosis. Many different methods and approaches are used for its treatment, which is also relevant for other acquired pathologies associated with loss of pigment or melanocyte function.

The book is intended for aestheticians, skincare specialists, dermatologists, specialists in aesthetic medicine, students at medical schools, and all interested persons.

ISBN 978-1-970196-29-0 (paperback)
ISBN 978-1-970196-04-7 (eBook — Adobe PDF)
ISBN 978-1-970196-28-3 (eBook — ePUB)

© Cosmetics & Medicine Publishing LLC, 2024
© Cover photo: Irina Bg / Shutterstock

FirstEditing

English version is edited and certified by the FirstEditing.Com, Inc. (USA).

Author/Editor

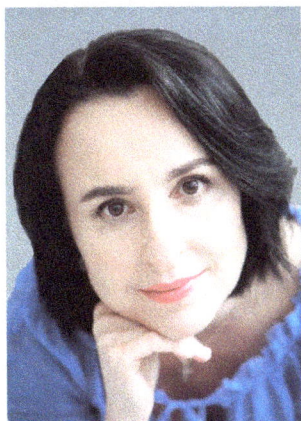

Elena I. Hernández-Jiménez, *Ph.D.*

Biophysicist, scientific journalist

Editor-in-chief of Cosmetics and Medicine Publishing

Chairperson of the Executive Board of the International Society of Applied Corneotherapy (I.A.C.)

Author and co-author of numerous publications in professional magazines, co-author and editor of the book series *Fundamentals of Cosmetic Dermatology & Skincare, Cosmetic Dermatology & Skincare Practice, Cosmetic Chemistry for Dermatology & Skincare Specialists* and others

Speaker at international conferences, author of training seminars and webinars for professionals in the field of skincare

Professional interests: biology and physiology of the skin, skin permeability, cosmetic chemistry, anti-age medicine, physiotherapy in dermatology and aesthetic medicine, skin analysis and imaging

Table of Contents

Abbreviations 10

Introduction 13

PART I
BIOLOGY & PHYSIOLOGY OF SKIN PIGMENTATION

Chapter 1. How pigmentation forms **15**
1.1. Skin color 15
1.2. Melanogenesis 16
    1.2.1. Melanocytes 17
    1.2.2. Stages of melanogenesis 21
        Melanin synthesis 21
        Pigment distribution in the epidermis 23
1.3. Melanin function. 24
1.4. Melanogenesis-regulating mechanisms 27

Chapter 2. Differences in skin pigmentation **30**
2.1. Skin phototypes 30
2.2. Ethnic skin types 33

Chapter 3. Pigmentation-affecting factors **37**
3.1. Hormones, stress, and inflammation 37
    3.1.1. Endocrine factors 37
    3.1.2. Inflammation. 38
    3.1.3. Stress 38
    3.1.4. Nutrient deficiencies 39
3.2. Solar radiation and tanning 40
    3.2.1. UV radiation 40
    3.2.2. Tanning. 43
        Immediate pigment darkening (IPD) 43
        Persistent pigment darkening (PPD) 44

3.3. Visible and infrared radiation 45

3.4. Air pollution 46

Chapter 4. Evolution of pigmentation:
adaptation to UV radiation 49

4.1. Internal "levers of pressure" in the evolution of pigmentation 50

    4.1.1. Why sunburn, cancer, and vitamin D overproduction
        are not evolutionary "levers" of pigmentation 50

    4.1.2. Folate is the key 52

    4.1.3. Vitamin D is the next candidate for the internal "lever"
        of natural selection 53

4.2. External force of natural selection: UV radiation 54

    4.2.1. Geographic variations of UV radiation 55

    4.2.2. UV as a driving force of selection
        in the pigmentation evolution 58

    4.2.3. UV radiation and the evolution of the skin's ability to tan 60

4.3. Conclusion 61

PART II

CLINICAL PICTURE & PIGMENTATION ANALYSIS

1.1. Pigmentation disorders 65

    1.1.1. Pigmentation disorders associated with an increase
        in the number of melanocytes 66

    Pigmented nevi 67

    Lentigo 67

    Peitz–Jeghers–Touraine syndrome 68

    Mongolian spot 68

    Nevus of Ota 68

    Nevus of Ito 68

    1.1.2. Pigmentation disorders associated with
        an increase in melanin 68

    Café-au-lait spots 69

    Freckles 69

    Melasma 69

Drug-induced pigmentation 70

Post-inflammatory pigmentation 71

Periorbital pigmentation 75

Phytophotodermatoses 76

Ashy dermatosis 76

1.1.3. Non-melanin-related skin color changes 76

Ochronosis 77

Argyria 77

Jaundice 77

1.1.4. Hypomelanoses 78

1.2. Pigmentation analysis 78

1.2.1. Anamnesis. 79

1.2.2. Examination 80

1.2.3. Instrumental evaluation of pigmentation when planning
aesthetic treatment 80

Mexametry 81

UV visualization 82

3D visualization 83

1.3. What pigmentation can an aesthetician work with? 84

PART III
AESTHETIC METHODS FOR PREVENTING
AND TREATING PIGMENT SPOTS

Chapter 1. Cosmetic products **91**

1.1. Depigmenting and lightening agents 91

1.1.1. Targets in the skin 91

1.1.2. Obsolete and dangerous substances 93

Mercury. 93

Phenol compounds 95

Hydroquinone. 95

1.1.3. Active substances in modern topical
pigmentation correctors 97

Azelaic acid 97

Arbutin 98

Kojic acid 99

Ascorbic acid 99

Niacinamide 100

N-acetylglycosamine 100

Tranexamic acid 100

Lignin peroxidase (lignase) 101

Cinnamic acid 101

Ferulic acid 101

Glycolic acid 102

Resveratrol 102

Fatty acids 103

1.1.4. Plant extracts with a complex lightening effect 103

Licorice 103

Soybean 104

Mulberry..104

Aloe 104

Green tea 105

Shiitake mushrooms 105

1.1.5. Retinoids 105

1.1.6. Whitening cosmetic formulations always contain
a combination of ingredients aimed at different targets 106

1.2. Sunscreens 107

1.2.1. UV filters 107

1.2.2. Protection against visible light 110

1.2.3. Safety..111

1.2.4. Requirements for sunscreen products 112

UVB protection: SPF — sun protection factor 114

UVA protection: PPD — persistent pigment darkening reaction..117

DNA PF — DNA protection factor 118

IPF — immune protection factor 118

1.2.5. Development of sunscreen formulation........................118

Combination of several UV filters — maximum protection
and minimum concentration 118

Product base — a guarantee of stability and
good textural properties 119

Substances with additional valuable properties 120

1.2.6. How to choose the correct sunscreen 121

1.3. Antioxidants 125

1.3.1. Natural antioxidants in cosmetic products 127

Vitamin E (tocopherol) 127

Vitamin C (L-ascorbic acid) 128

β-Carotene 128

α-Lipoic acid (thioctic acid) 128

Coenzyme Q_{10} (ubiquinone) 128

Antioxidant herbal compositions 129

1.3.2. The art of antioxidant formulation 130

1.3.3. Selection algorithm for antioxidant skincare products 132

Antioxidant composition (primary antioxidant protection) 132

Protection of antioxidants against oxidation and degradation
(secondary antioxidant protection) 135

1.4. Cosmetic camouflage 136

**Chapter 2. Energy-based technologies for
treating pigmentation disorders** **137**

2.1. Light therapy 137

2.1.1. Skin preparation for laser treatment 137

2.1.2. Mechanism of action 138

2.1.3. Light technologies for treating pigmentary lesions 140

Green light 142

Yellow light 143

Red light 144

Near-IR light 144

Intensive pulse light (IPL) 145

Laser resurfacing and fractional photothermolysis 146

2.1.4. Low-level laser radiation 148

2.1.5. Effectiveness of laser treatment in pigmentation
disorders 149

2.2. Mechanical methods 151

2.2.1. Microdermabrasion 151

2.2.2. Gas–liquid microdermabrasion 152

Chapter 3. Injectable methods **154**

3.1. Microneedling 154

3.2. Biorevitalization 156

3.3. PRP therapy 157

Chapter 4. Nutraceuticals for skin lightening **158**

4.1. Glutathione 158

4.2. *Polypodium leucotomos* fern extract 159

4.3. Tranexamic acid 160

PART IV

VITILIGO

1.1. Light therapy.. 163

    1.1.1. Narrow band UVB (311 nm) 163

    1.1.2. Focused microphototherapy (Bioskin Evolution®)............... 163

    1.1.3. B-band (XeCl) narrow-band UVB (308 nm) excimer laser 164

    1.1.4. PUVA therapy 164

    1.1.5. Photodynamic therapy.. 164

    1.1.6. Sunscreens 165

1.2. Pharmacotherapy 166

1.3. Cosmetic and nutraceutical ingredients 167

1.4. Surgical methods 168

1.5. Depigmentation 168

1.6. Cosmetic camouflage.. 169

1.7. Treatment efficacy and prognosis 169

Conclusion **170**

References **172**

Abbreviations

6H5MICA — 6-hydroxy-5-methoxy-indole-2-carboxylic acid

7-DHC — 7-dehydrocholesterol

ACTH — adrenocorticotropic hormone

AHA — alpha hydroxy acid

AhR — aryl hydrocarbon receptors

ALA — aminolevulinic acid

ATP — adenosine triphosphate

bFGF — basic fibroblast growth factor

BH4 — tetrahydrobiopterin

BHA — butylated hydroxyanisole

BHT — butylated hydroxytoluene

BMP-4 — bone morphogenetic protein

cAMP — cyclic adenosine mono-phosphate

CGRP — calcitonin gene-related peptide

CNS — central nervous system

CPD — cyclobutane pyrimidine dimer

CV — coefficient of variation

DHA — dihydroxyacetone

DHI — 5,6-dihydroxyindole

DHICA — 5,6-dihydroxyindole-2-carboxylic acid

DKK1 — Dickkopf 1 protein

DNA — deoxyribonucleic acid

DNA PF — DNA protection factor

DOPA — L-3,4-dioxyphenylalanine

ECGC — epigallo-catechin-3-gal-late

EDN — endothelin

EDTA — ethylenediaminetetra-acetic acid

EGF — epidermal growth factor

Er:glass — erbium glass laser

Er:YAG — erbium-doped yttrium aluminum garnet laser

Er:YSGG — erbium, chromium, yttrium, scandium, gallium garnet laser

ET-1 — endothelin 1

FDA — U.S. Food and Drug Administration

FGF — fibroblast growth factor

GM-CSF — granulocyte-macrophage colony-stimulating factor

GTP — guanosine triphosphate

HA — hyaluronic acid

HGF — hepatocyte growth factor

hGH — human growth hormone (somatotropin)

HPA — hypothalamic-pituitary-adrenal

HS — heparan sulfate

IFN	— interferon	NASA	— National Aeronautics and Space Administration
IL	— interleukin		
INCI	— International Nomenclature of Cosmetic Ingredients	Nd:YAG	— neodymium-doped yttrium aluminum garnet laser
IPD	— immediate pigment darkening	NGF	— nerve growth factor
		NO	— nitric oxide
IPL	— intense pulsed light	NRG-1	— neuregulin-1
IPT	— individual protection time	NSAID	— non-steroidal anti-inflammatory drug
IR	— infrared light		
IUDs	— intrauterine devices	NTDs	— neural tube defects
JAK	— Janus kinase inhibitors	OPN3	— opsin-3 receptor
KGF	— keratinocyte growth factor	PABA	— para-aminobenzoic acid
KTP	— potassium titanyl phos-phate laser	PAH	— polycyclic aromatic hydrocarbon
		PDGF	— platelet-derived growth factor
LED	— light emitting diode	PDL	— pulsed dye laser
LIF	— leukemia inhibitory factor	PDT	— photodynamic therapy
LLLT	— low-level laser therapy	PG	— prostaglandin
		PGE2	— prostaglandin E2
MAL	— methyl ester of ALA	PGF2α	— prostaglandin F2α
MC1R	— melanocortin-1 receptor	PM	— particulate matter
MED	— minimal erythema dose	POMC	— pro-opiomelanocortin
MITF	— microphthalmia-associat-ed transcription factor	PPD	— persistent pigment darkening
MMP	— matrix metalloproteinase	PRP	— platelet-rich plasma
MSH	— melanocyte-stimulating hormone	PTN	— pleiotrophin
		PUVA	— psoralen and UVA
MTHF	— 5-methyltetrahydrofolate		
MTZ	— microthermal zones	QS	— Q-Switched
MC1R	— melanocortin-1 receptor		
		RF	— radiofrequency
NADPH	— nicotinamide adenine dinucleotide phosphate (abbreviated NADP+); NADPH is the reduced form of NADP+	RNA	— ribonucleic acid
		ROS	— reactive oxygen species
		SASP	— senescence-associated secretory phenotype

SBEG — suction blister epidermal grafts

SCF — stem cell factor

sFRP2 — secreted frizzle-related protein-2

SP — substance P

SPF — sun protection factor

TGF — transforming growth factor

TNF — tumor necrosis factor

TRPs — transient receptor potential ion channels

TRT — thermal relaxation time

TSH — thyroid stimulating hormone (thyrotropin, thyrotrophin)

TYR — tyrosinase

TYRP — tyrosinase-related protein

UV — ultraviolet

UVA — ultraviolet type A

UVB — ultraviolet type B

UVC — ultraviolet type C

VEGF — vascular endothelial growth factor

VIP — vasoactive intestinal peptide

Introduction

The color of our skin is one of the main outward characteristics distinguishing people from each other. Although skin color depends on many factors, the pigment melanin is the main one. The amount of melanin determines whether the skin is light and easily burns in the sun or has a photodamage-resistant, chocolate-like hue. Although the skin of a healthy person — regardless of race — is fairly evenly colored, there are conditions in which the distribution of melanin can be disturbed for various reasons.

These conditions fall into two broad groups: **hyperpigmentation** conditions, which are associated with brown or gray–blue spots, and **hypopigmentation** disorders, which appear as discoloration of some skin regions. Although neither the former nor the latter usually threaten health and are aesthetic defects, their presence can cause considerable anxiety. Not surprisingly, people are willing to spend a lot of effort to correct them. Although psychological work is also very important here, cosmetic help can significantly improve the quality of life for people with pigmentary disorders.

Skincare specialists can do a lot to help. Over the past decades, we have learned much about the mechanisms of pigmentation formation and its causes, studied many new therapeutic agents that are much safer than their predecessors, and developed technologies for selective action on pigment. We have also learned that combating pigmentation is a complex step-by-step process that requires time, careful implementation of recommendations, and patience from both the patient and the specialist. Still, it is a story that can have a happy ending.

In this book, we have gathered all the information you need to understand the intricacies of pigmentation lesion formation, which is important for drawing up an effective and safe aesthetic treatment program. It is intended primarily for specialists — beauticians, aestheticians, skincare specialists, dermatologists — but it will provide answers for everyone interested in skincare and treatment of pigment lesions. So, let's begin!

Part I

Biology & physiology of skin pigmentation

Chapter 1
How pigmentation forms

1.1. Skin color

Color is a qualitative characteristic of any visible object. However, the **color** we see in most cases is not the **light** that the object emits by itself but rather the part of the visible spectrum that this object reflects. When light strikes an object, some of that light is absorbed by it, and some of it is scattered so that only the remaining reflected part will be visible to the observer (**Fig. I-1-1**). Thanks to the reflected light, we see objects in color (depending on what part of the visible spectrum it has reflected, as in the rainbow — from violet to red).

Skin contains several chromophore pigments that absorb radiation and cause skin color (**Fig. I-1-2**). These include:

- Melanin
- Hemoglobin (oxy- and deoxyhemoglobin)
- Lipofuscin
- Bilirubin
- Carotenoids

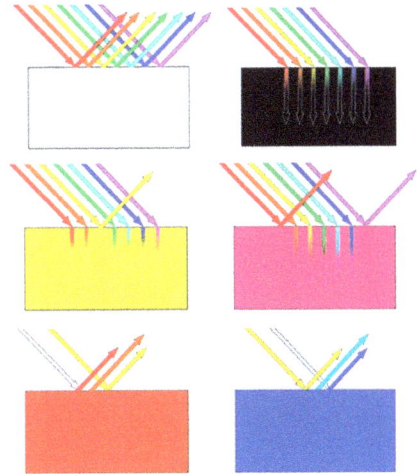

Figure I-1-1. The color of the object we see is due to the processes of absorption and reflection of different parts of the visible light spectrum

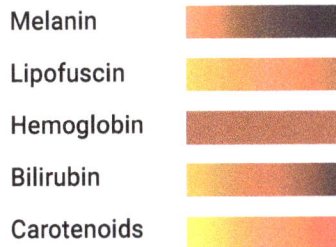

Melanin

Lipofuscin

Hemoglobin

Bilirubin

Carotenoids

Figure I-1-2. Skin pigments coloring the skin

Apart from "coloring substances," the shine and brightness of our skin color depend on the condition of its surface (smooth or rough), the thickness of its individual layers, and the condition of the vascular bed (distribution, number, and condition of blood vessels). Oxygenated hemoglobin in capillaries and arterioles gives the skin a pink or reddish tone, and the venous network has a bluish tint. Young people suffering from vegetative neurosis often have a scarlet face, causing them a lot of suffering. In some diseases, dilated blood vessels stain the cheeks, nose, and chin with a bluish–red color.

The *stratum corneum* is heterogeneous, and that, too, contributes to skin tone. Sometimes to improve your complexion, it's enough to clean up the *stratum corneum* by exfoliating old flakes and smoothing out its surface. Skin tone is also affected by the water content of the *stratum corneum*. Skin appears brighter when the *stratum corneum* is saturated with water. Even subcutaneous fat can affect skin tone, especially when the epidermis and dermis are thinning (for example, after a serious illness). In this case, the skin takes on a characteristic yellowish hue (Piña-Oviedo S. et al., 2017).

So many factors influence skin color, but melanin is undoubtedly the most important one because it is the base color. Its contribution, even in white people rarely exposed to the sun, is quite significant, as you can easily see by looking at the skin of vitiligo patients — areas of skin lacking melanin are very prominent (**Fig. I-1-3**).

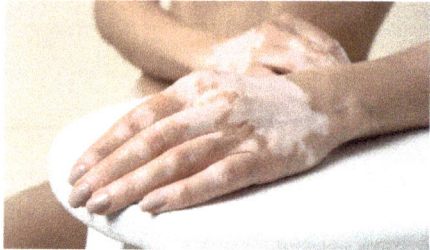

Figure I-1-3. Vitiligo (Image by Freepik.com)

The distribution of melanin in the skin is the most variable phenotypic trait and the main factor determining the diversity of the human population.

1.2. Melanogenesis

Skin melanin pigmentation is divided into **constitutive**, fixed genetically (it determines the skin phenotype), and **facultative**, caused by external or internal influences. Optional pigmentation is divided into physiological (tanning) and pathological (e.g., post-inflammatory pigmentation caused by hormonal imbalances, solar lentigo). Of course, constitutive pigmentation is also physiological.

Many cells and signaling pathways are involved in pigmentation formation. Still, the main ones are melanocytes and keratinocytes, which carry out the processes of pigment formation (melanogenesis) and distribution in the skin. Melanocytes are connected by protein bridges (desmosomes) with the basal membrane, surrounding keratinocytes, and each other. Together they form a single functional unit, in which one melanocyte forms connections with 36 (from 30 to 40) keratinocytes on average. This structure is called the **epidermal melanin unit** (some authors suggest considering the participation of Langerhans cells in these close relations) (Bauer J. et al., 2001; Nordlund J.J., 2007). Surprisingly, this balance is maintained throughout human life, although we still do not fully understand how exactly (Thingnes J. et al., 2012).

1.2.1. Melanocytes

Melanin synthesis is carried out by melanocytes, large dendritic cells located in the basal layer of the epidermis (**Fig. I-1-4**). Three types of melanocytes are found in human skin:

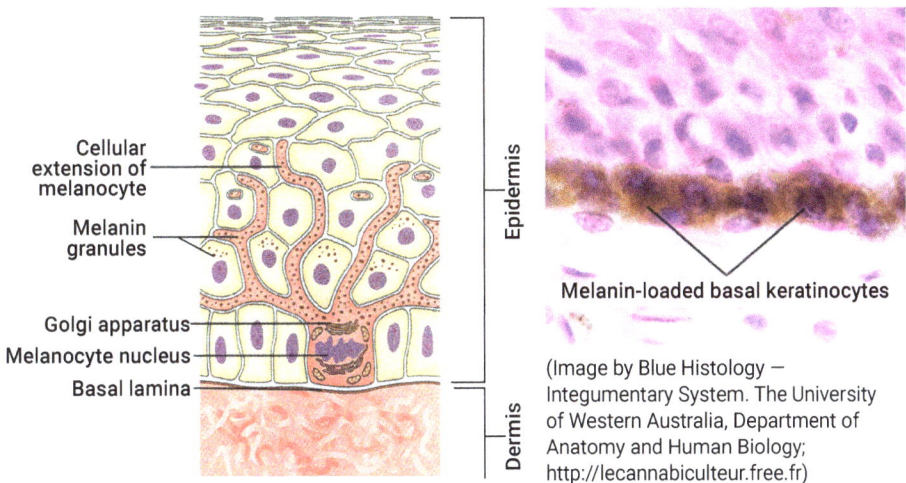

Melanin-loaded basal keratinocytes

(Image by Blue Histology — Integumentary System. The University of Western Australia, Department of Anatomy and Human Biology; http://lecannabiculteur.free.fr)

Figure I-1-4. Melanin and keratinocytes form a functional unit

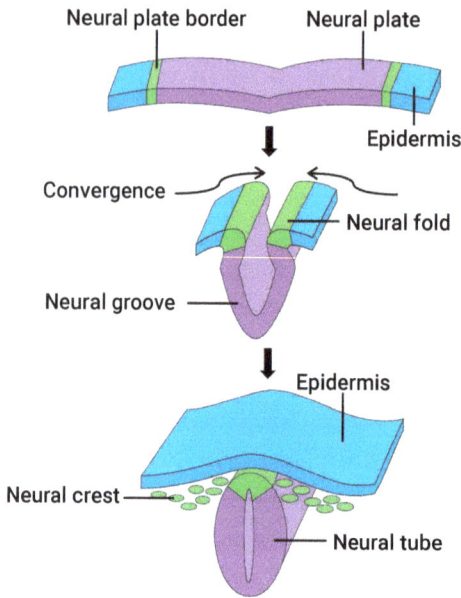

Figure I-1-5.
The formation of neural crest during the process of neurulation
(Image by Wikipedia.com)

1. Light bipolar cells (they are less differentiated than other melanocytes and contain no pigment)
2. Melanocytes in hair follicles
3. Epidermal melanocytes

During embryonic development, melanocytes do not reach their permanent dislocation sites immediately. Initially, all epidermal and nerve cells develop from the same embryo — ectoderm. However, if the pathways of keratinocytes and nerve cells diverge quite early, melanocyte precursors (melanoblasts) still develop for some time within the neural crest (**Fig. I-1-5**). Only by 6–8 weeks of intrauterine development do they "catch up" with the epithelial (outer) ectoderm, penetrating the basal layer of epidermis and hair follicle buds (it is assumed they use the nerve endings growing into the skin as a "funicular" for this). By weeks 12–13, most of them are found in the epidermis and hair follicles (a little later), where they differentiate into melanocytes. Some melanoblasts do not differentiate and are "stored" in the bulge of the hair follicle as fission-capable stem cells. There is an assumption that some of them can remain directly in the dermis (Bismuth K. et al., 2017).

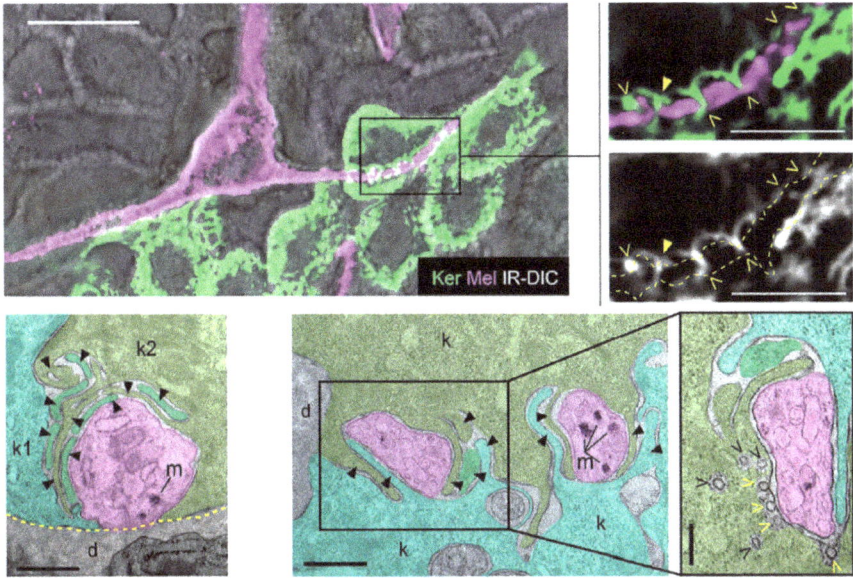

Figure I-1-6. Contacts formed between keratinocytes (green staining) and melanocytes (pink staining). Data obtained through immunofluorescence and transmission electron microscopy (adapted from Belote R.L., Simon S.M., 2020)

Differentiated melanocytes, fixed to the basal membrane, begin to grow dendrites — outgrowths by which they communicate with keratinocytes and transfer the formed melanosomes containing melanin to them. Melanocytes can lengthen their dendrites when needed (e.g., intensive insolation, damage), "turning" towards the source of "help" signals. Thus, although melanocytes are referred to as skin cells, they retain even their external resemblance to neurons.

However, not only melanocytes show affinity to the nervous system. A study published in 2020 by Belote R.L. and Simon S.M. showed that keratinocytes also have microscopic outgrowths of cytoplasm with which they "embrace" melanocyte dendrites, resembling the arrangement of glial cells of the nervous system (**Fig. I-1-6**). Moreover, it turned out that keratinocytes and melanocytes "communicate" with each other not only with the help of signal molecules common for skin, which will be discussed later, but also neurotransmitters, in particular acetylcholine (Belote R.L., Simon S.M., 2020). Articles published by Prof. L. Misery, a world-renowned expert on skin sensitivity, further demonstrate that there are sensitive receptors (transient receptor potential ion channels, TRPs) on the surface of keratinocytes, the same ones that are found on free nerve endings (Tagalas M., Misery L., 2019).

According to different sources, the ratio of melanocytes to keratinocytes in the basal layer varies from 1:4 to 1:10 depending on the area of the body — primarily the area exposed to or protected from ultraviolet (UV) rays. The ratio of melanocytes to keratinocytes in the photoprotected areas may decrease with age — they slowly migrate to offer a "helping hand" to their counterparts in the areas that need intensive sun protection. This (among other factors) explains why even light-skinned people burn less in the sun than they did while growing up (Alaluf S. et al., 2002; Alaluf S. et al., 2003; Thingnes J. et al., 2012). However, such "battles," as well as other injuries, can lead to melanocyte death. In general, after the age of 30, the number of melanocytes decreases by about 10–20% every decade. It should be noted that the exact lifespan of epidermal melanocytes is currently unknown, although it is very long. However, hair follicle melanocytes live only for about 3–5 years (Tobin D.J., 2011).

Interestingly, because of their long lifespan, melanocytes have recently been "blamed" for epidermal aging. A study conducted by Victorelli S. et al. published in late 2019 showed that aging (senescent) melanocytes are the only epidermal cell type that expresses the aging marker p16[INK4A]. The problem is that, as they age, like dermal fibroblasts, melanocytes acquire a senescence-associated secretory phenotype (SASP). This phenotype ("lifestyle") is associated with releasing many factors into the extracellular environment, causing inflammation and destructive changes in the extracellular matrix, negatively affecting the activity of the remaining epidermal cells. Thus, senescent melanocytes have been shown to disrupt basal keratinocyte proliferation and promote epidermal atrophy *in vitro* (Victorelli S. et al., 2019).

Melanocytes are found in the epidermis, hair papilla, and iris. The pigment they produce gives color to the hair and eyes. If there is a lot of melanin, the eyes are brown; if there is little, they are blue, and the combination of a small amount of melanin and lipofuscin gives the eyes a green color.

Besides, melanocytes are present in the inner ear in part of the cochlear duct wall, presumably regulating the ionic composition of the endolymph and ensuring the proper functioning of auditory hair cells. It has been suggested that a decrease in the number of melanocytes can lead to hearing impairment — such as in Waardenburg syndrome, characterized by pigment abnormalities of the skin, hair, and eyes as well as varying degrees of deafness or albinism, which can also be accompanied by hearing impairment. However, the function of melanocytes when involved in regulating hearing does not depend on their ability to produce pigment because mammals that lack melanin but retain melanocytes usually have normal hearing. Consequently, melanocytes play an important role beyond that associated with pigmentation. We now know that melanocytes are found in the inner ear, nervous system, and heart, but this is likely not the end of the list. However, melanin synthesis in these organs is not their primary function (Cichorek M. et al., 2013).

1.2.2. Stages of melanogenesis

Melanin synthesis

Melanin is synthesized in melanocytes from the amino acid tyrosine in a series of sequential oxidative reactions. The first two stages of this process, the conversion of tyrosine to dioxyphenylalanine (DOPA) quinone via DOPA, are carried out with the participation of the enzyme tyrosinase. Tyrosinase is a copper-containing oxidase produced only by melanocytes. It catalyzes the oxidation of phenolic compounds, including tyrosine. Its synthesis and "maturation" occur in the endoplasmic network and Golgi apparatus, after which tyrosinase is sent to melanosomes, where it is stored in a membrane-bound state.

DOPA-quinone is then converted to DOPA-chrome containing an indole ring, from which the colorless dihydroxyindole-2-carboxylic acid (5,6-dihydroxyindole-2-carboxylic acid, DHICA) is synthesized by DOPA-chrome tautomerase (also known as tyrosinase-related protein 2, or TYRP2) in the presence of metal ions. The products of DHICA oxidation — enzymatic (involving TYRP1) or non-enzymatic — polymerize to form brown DHICA melanin, which includes 100 to 1000 DHICA monomers.

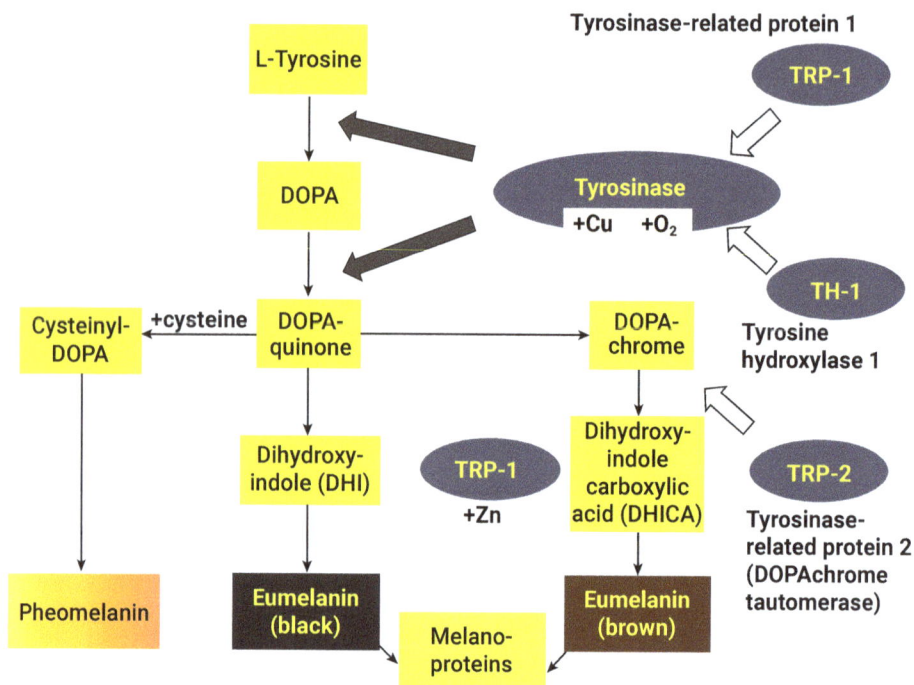

Figure I-1-7. Melanin biosynthesis

DOPA-chrome can also be converted to 5,6-dihydroxyindole (DHI). The product of oxidative polymerization of DHI is black DHI melanin (**Fig. I-1-7**). Peroxidase and DHICA-oxidase enzymes are involved in the polymerization of DHICA and DHI.

DHI and DHICA are called **eumelanin** and are black–brown in color. They are the main type of skin melanin.

In addition, in the presence of glutathione or cysteine in melanocytes, cysteinyl-DOPA (5-S-cysteinyl-DOPA) is formed from DOPA-quinone, which when polymerized leads to the formation of a lighter pigment, **pheomelanin** (yellow–red color).

Both eumelanin and pheomelanin are always formed during melanogenesis but in different ratios. These ratios are determined by tyrosinase activity and tyrosine and cysteine concentrations in the substrate as well as, generally, by the genetic programming.

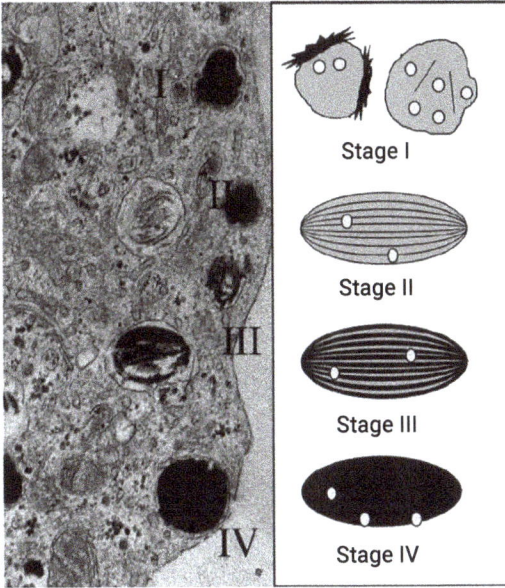

Figure I-1-8. Stages of melanosome development. Tyrosinase "attaches" to immature melanosomes in the second stage of their development. From this moment, the direct process of melanin synthesis begins (adapted from Raposo G., Marks M.S., 2002).

Pigment distribution in the epidermis

Melanin synthesizes and accumulates in melanosomes, organelles surrounded by a membrane. This process occurs because melanosomes isolate melanogenesis from the rest of the cell and prevent the toxic effect of reactive melanin intermediates. Melanosomes undergo several stages of development (I–IV), characterized by the formation of a microfilament network and the accumulation of synthesized melanin at various degrees of maturity (**Fig. I-1-8**). Mature melanosomes containing eumelanin are ellipsoidal, while those containing pheomelanin are spherical (Raposo G., Marks M.S., 2002).

As melanin matures, melanosomes move from the central part of the melanocyte to its offshoots, where they "anchor" to the microtubular system. They are pulled up by actin and myosin to the dendrites' end sections and sent to keratinocytes. How melanosomes are transferred to keratinocytes is still unclear — different studies indicate different mechanisms: membrane fusion, phagocytosis, vesicular transfer, cytophagocytosis.

After melanosomes enter the keratinocyte, they accumulate around the nuclei in the form of so-called melanin caps protecting the main organelle of the cell — the nucleus — from damage by UV light and

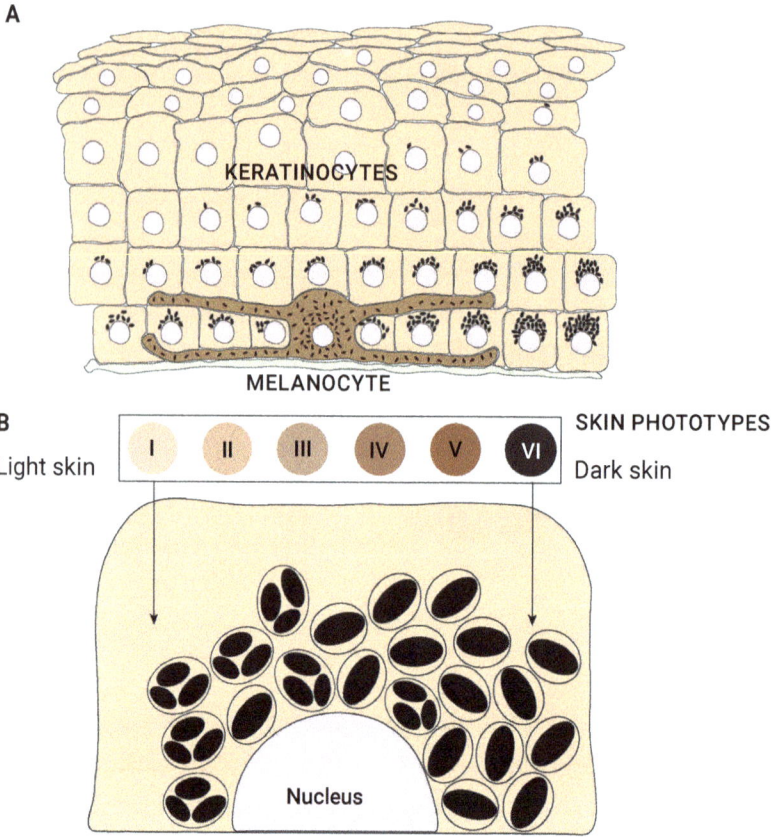

Figure I-1-9. Melanin distribution throughout the epidermis (A) and organization within keratinocytes (B) (adapted from Bento-Lopes L. et al., 2023)

other factors (**Fig. I-1-9**). Further, melanin-laden keratinocytes migrate upward and, in the case of epithelialization after injury, to the sides. Thus, the melanin "umbrella" opens over the entire epidermis.

1.3. Melanin function

It was originally thought that the main function of melanin in human skin was to regulate the amount of UV radiation penetrating the skin, i.e., to serve as a UV filter. Once sunlight hits the skin, melanocytes are activated and work harder to saturate the epidermis with more melanin and strengthen the "sun umbrella" (Baldea I. et al., 2009). The skin darkens — it becomes tanned. The resulting tan does not disappear immediately after cessation of exposure to UV and is visible until the keratinocytes, loaded with excess melanin, naturally leave the epidermis.

Indeed, both eumelanin and pheomelanin actively absorb UV radiation. However, when they absorb it, they behave like any other molecule—they try to get rid of extra energy somehow. Part of the energy turns into heat, and part of it is spent on photochemical reactions that form free radicals. This is a problem because melanin can increase skin damage by generating additional radicals to those already formed under the influence of UV.

However, eumelanin, in addition to its ability to absorb UV light, is a trap for free radicals, i.e., an antioxidant. It is large and stable enough to independently utilize the formed reactive oxygen species (ROS) (Bustamante J. et al., 1993).

In recent years, the colorless melanin precursors DHI and DHICA have also become the object of intensive research. The findings indicate that their role in the skin is no less important than that of black and brown melanin. In particular, DHI and DHICA inhibit peroxidation reactions, supporting the functioning of melanocyte antioxidant systems (Pellosi M.C. et al., 2014). They have even been suggested for inclusion in cosmetics— as antioxidants, sunscreens, and visible light filters (Panzella L. et al., 2018). However, the potential for using mature melanin for this purpose is also actively investigated (Solano F., 2014).

Pheomelanin, on the other hand, does not "behave" so well. The sulfhydryl bonds in cysteine, the amino acid that gives it its characteristic red–yellow color, are prone to oxidation, reducing pheomelanin's stability. Its "antioxidant power" is insufficient to effectively neutralize radicals produced after UV light exposure. Moreover, other melanocyte antioxidants, including glutathione, the first-line antioxidant, are sent to fight these radicals. As a result, the "rear" is left uncovered, and the melanocyte antioxidant systems are depleted. They are also depleted because glutathione is used to synthesize pheomelanin to compensate for "combat losses." In addition, the amount of nicotinamide adenine dinucleotide phosphate (NADPH) decreases, and the oxidation of melanin precursors increases (Panzella L. et al., 2014).

Research further shows that dysplastic nevi, a known risk factor for melanoma, have higher levels of pheomelanin, which produces large amounts of ROS and leads to more pronounced oxidative deoxyribonucleic acid (DNA) damage than in melanocytes from normal skin of the same donor (Smit N.P. et al., 2008). Moreover, some authors have documented oxidative DNA damage in the presence of pheomelanin, even without exposure to UV or some other damaging factor (Panzella L. et al., 2018). In addition, it has been suggested that pheomelanin degradation under the influence of ultraviolet type A (UVA) radiation can lead to the formation of DNA mutations called cyclobutane pyrimidine dimers (CPDs), previously thought to be specific for ultraviolet type B (UVB) exposure (see Part I, section 3.2 for details on the UV effects). These UVA-induced dimers are called "dark" because they form after UV exposure ceases (Delinasios G.J. et al., 2018).

Recently, it has become clear that the role of melanin is not limited to the absorption of UV radiation. Today, melanin (except for pheomelanin) is ascribed the following biological functions:

- **Photoprotective and radioprotective** — absorb quanta of ionizing, UV radiation, and visible light
- **Antioxidant** — eumelanin and its precursors can neutralize free radicals, ROS, and other active oxygen-containing compounds
- **Buffer** — melanin is a redox polymer that buffers the level of other intracellular redox biomolecules
- **Chelating** — melanin can bind many metal ions with high efficiency (thus, they can isolate potentially toxic metal ions, protecting the rest of the cell from them)
- **Detoxifying** — these polymers have a pronounced ability to bind various organic molecules, xenobiotics, aromatic and lipophilic compounds
- **Thermoregulatory** — capable of dissipating up to 90% of the absorbed solar energy in the form of heat
- **Presentational** — interface characteristics provided by melanin in the skin, hair, and eyes

Research conducted in recent decades has shown that melanocytes contribute significantly to the skin's response to almost **any stressor**, working in conjunction with the skin's neuroimmune system. Thus, the traditional view of melanocytes as cells responsible for skin color and protection from sunburn has given way to a more complex and interesting concept, i.e., melanocytes are sensors of skin stressors.

Another important point is the established connection between melanogenesis and redox processes. This indicates a close interaction of photoprotective mechanisms with the second line of defense of the skin, including the immune and antioxidant systems.

1.4. Melanogenesis-regulating mechanisms

In fish, amphibians, and reptiles, melanogenesis is under the control of pituitary hormones. In general, this process looks as follows: light hits the photoreceptors, from them comes a signal to the brain, then the pituitary gland starts producing melanocyte-stimulating hormone (MSH). In response to MSH, melanosomes move from the body of the melanocyte to the sponges, causing the skin to darken. After some time, the melanosomes move back, and the skin becomes lighter again. MSH is found in all animals (humans are no exception), but its involvement in changes in human skin pigmentation is not as apparent as in lower vertebrates.

In humans, melanogenesis is regulated at the systemic and local levels.

At the **systemic** level, the following systems are involved:

- Endocrine system — hormones of the hypothalamus, pituitary gland, adrenal glands, sex glands, and thyroid have a stimulating effect; epiphysis hormone (melatonin) has an inhibitory effect
- Autonomic nervous system — sympathetic (noradrenaline) stimulates, parasympathetic (acetylcholine) inhibits melanogenesis
- Central nervous system (CNS; see Part I, section 3.1)

The pituitary hormones — melanocyte-stimulating (MSH) and adrenocorticotropic (ACTH) hormones — play the main role. There are several types of MSH — alpha, beta, and gamma, and they affect not only pigmentation. The main type that directly regulates melanin synthesis and secretion is α-MSH. It affects melanocytes through a special receptor for melanocyte-stimulating hormone, MC1R, on the cell surface. MC1R is also sensitive to ACTH. Both these hormones, α-MSH and ACTH, are cleavage products of pro-opiomelanocortin (POMC). Their binding to melanocytes initiates a complex signaling cascade that leads to the production of eumelanin.

However, the main role in regulating melanogenesis in humans is played not by pituitary α-MSH but by the keratinocytes of the epidermis directly produced under the influence of UV radiation and other damaging factors. It should be said that the exact mechanisms that control the organization, number, and activity of melanocytes in the epidermis are still being studied.

Keratinocytes, dermal fibroblasts, immune cells, nerve endings, and components of the extracellular matrix — that is, all structural components of the skin — communicate with melanocytes (and each other) via many signaling molecules, thus informing melanocytes of some dangers and regulating pigmentation **locally**. Keratinocytes and fibroblasts are a local source of hormones and active compounds that regulate melanocyte proliferation, melanogenesis, and melanocyte dendrite formation. Under stress influences, free nerve endings produce various neuropeptides, e.g., neuropeptides encoded by the calcitonin gene, substance P (SP), which also stimulate melanogenesis. For details on the CNS influence on the skin (stress mechanisms), see Part I, section 3.1.

Melanin synthesis also enhances nitric oxide (NO) production by activated macrophages, which explains why UVB-induced pigmentation occurs after erythema. NO-induced vasodilation is an important link in the pathogenesis of UVB-induced erythema. At the same time, increased nitric oxide levels are observed in any inflammatory response (Yuan X.H., Jin Z.H., 2018). The crosstalk of different signaling pathways between these cells is part of the system that maintains skin homeostasis. We won't go into the molecular details, but **Fig. I-1-10** provides the basic elements of this truly active signaling communication (Yuan X.H., Jin S.H., 2018).

It turns out that melanocytes "hear" the cries of help from practically any skin inhabitant (and not only skin), even if they are not addressed directly to them. In response, melanocytes activate or inhibit melanogenesis, outgrowth formation (dendritogenesis), and melano-

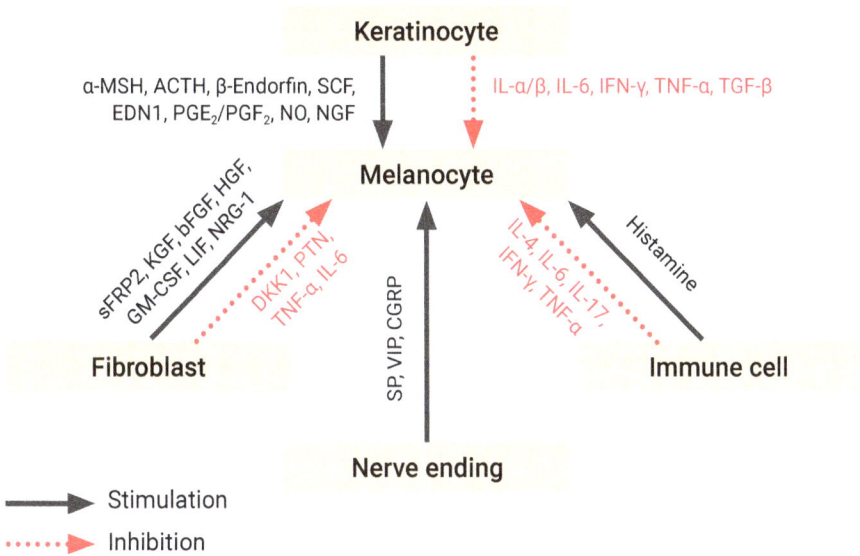

Figure I-1-10. Signals sent by keratinocytes, fibroblasts, immune cells, and nerve endings to the melanocyte in response to stress exposure (UV, pollutants, etc.)

Abbreviations: α-MSH — alpha melanocyte-stimulating hormone; ACTH — adrenocorticotropic hormone; SCF — stem cell factor; EDN1 — endothelin 1; NO — nitric oxide; NGF — nerve growth factor; PGE_2 /PGF_2 — prostaglandins; sFRP2 — secreted frizzle-related protein-2; KGF — keratinocyte growth factor; bFGF — basic fibroblast growth factor; HGF — hepatocyte growth factor; GM-CSF — granulocyte-macrophage colony-stimulating factor; LIF — leukemia inhibitory factor; NRG-1 — neuregulin-1; DKK1 — Dickkopf 1 protein; PTN — pleiotrophin; IL — interleukin; IFN — interferon; TNF — tumor necrosis factor; TGF — transforming growth factor; CGRP — calcitonin gene-related peptide; SP — substance P; VIP — vasoactive intestinal peptide.

some transport activity, or slow down their life path (activation and inhibition of proliferation and differentiation) and even die.

Thus, we can say that **melanogenesis should be increased by any exposure where cell damage, ROS generation, and immune system activation occur**. In other words, triggering melanogenesis is part of the skin's universal response to any stressful exposure, not just UV exposure, as previously thought. This explains many clinical observations, particularly the appearance of pigmentation in the absence of UV exposure (e.g., post-inflammatory, post-traumatic, hormonal diseases).

Chapter 2
Differences in skin pigmentation

2.1. Skin phototypes

People across the planet have different skin colors, ranging from very light beige to almost black. Currently, there is no universally accepted classification of skin phototypes. The earlier classifications, based on outward appearance — skin color, eye color, hair color — do not adequately assess the wide range of variants resulting from mixing genotypes of representatives of different races.

The main classification currently used by most specialists is the slightly modified version of the classification developed by the American dermatologist Thomas Fitzpatrick in 1975. It is based on the response of the different skin types to UV radiation, i.e., the skin's ability to tan, and reflects well the distribution by skin color in general. Fitzpatrick scale includes six phototypes (**Fig. I-2-1**):

I. Celtic — skin never tans, always burns (very light skin, blond or red hair, blue or green eyes, freckles)

II. Light-skinned Caucasian — sometimes manages to tan, but more often burns (light skin, blond or brown hair, blue, green, or gray eyes)

III. Dark-skinned Caucasian — skin tans well but sometimes burns (medium shade of skin from light to swarthy, dark brown or brown hair, usually brown eyes)

IV. Mediterranean/Asian — skin tans quickly, rarely burns (light brown skin, dark brown or brown hair, usually brown eyes)

V. Hindu — skin never burns (very dark skin, black hair, black eyes)

VI. African — skin never burns (dark skin, black hair, black eyes)

Concerning UV irradiation, phototypes I and II are considered melanin deficient (no protection), phototypes III and IV are melanocompetent

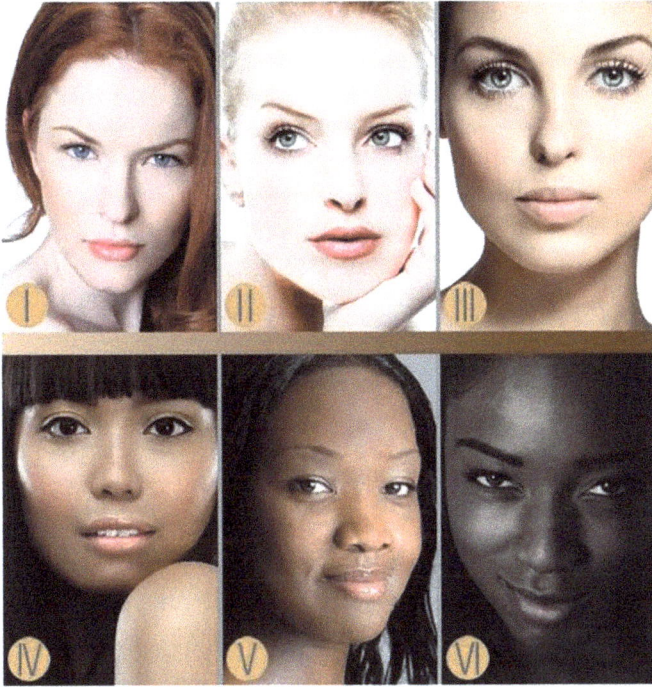

Figure I-2-1. Fitzpatrick skin phototypes

(acquired protection), and phototypes V and VI are melanin protective (innate protection).

In some individuals, it is impossible to detect a skin reaction due to the high degree of pigmentation.

Fitzpatrick's classification is simple and accessible, which is convenient when working with patients, but it does not consider the full variety of skin colors. Color can be determined more accurately using the **anthropological chromatic scale of von Luschan** (Felix von Luschan, 1854–1924), a German anthropologist who suggested identifying all possible skin color variations by comparing it to 36 glass reference color plates. To avoid bias, measurements are made by applying the reference plate to the inner side of the forearm of the examinee. This method gives excellent accuracy in determining skin color and is still used in anthropology but is not common in dermatology.

The **Lancer Ethnic Scale** (H.A. Lancer), proposed in 1998, allows us to specify the phototype by considering heredity. The phototypes

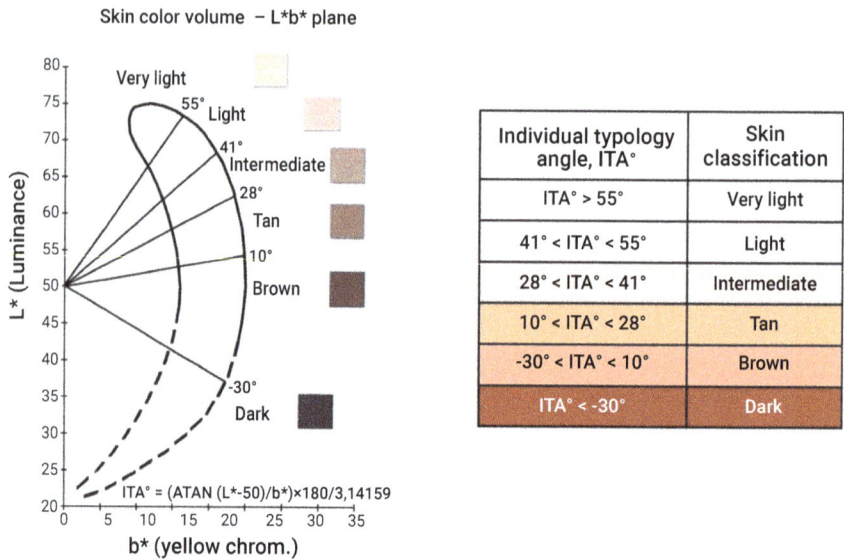

Skin color volume – L*b* plane

Individual typology angle, ITA°	Skin classification
ITA° > 55°	Very light
41° < ITA° < 55°	Light
28° < ITA° < 41°	Intermediate
10° < ITA° < 28°	Tan
-30° < ITA° < 10°	Brown
ITA° < -30°	Dark

Figure I-2-2. Integral characterization of skin color using spectrophotometry (adapted from Del Bino S., Bernerd F., 2013)

(according to Fitzpatrick) of both sets of grandparents are summed and divided by four. This refinement allows us to anticipate some side effects of light cosmetic procedures (Lancer H.A., 1998).

An integral characteristic of skin color is currently provided by **colorimetric methods** (Del Bino S., Bernerd F., 2013). Using a spectrophotometer, the reflected light in the visible part of the spectrum (400–700 nm) is measured, and the following parameters are determined (**Fig. I-2-2**):

- L* (brightness)
- a* and b* (green–red and blue–yellow chromatic coordinates)
- °ITA (individual typological angle, pigmentation intensity)
- C* (color saturation)
- h* (hue)

The integral characteristic of skin color is used mainly in scientific research, while in practice the Fitzpatrick phototype assessment remains popular.

2.2. Ethnic skin types

If we consider skin color in a young person without skin disease, it will be remarkably uniform regardless of race. The main reason for that is the uniform distribution of melanocytes over the whole basal layer of the epidermis — as we mentioned before, the ratio of keratinocytes and melanocytes in the basal layer is constant — ranging from 1:4 to 1:10 in different parts of the body. Melanocyte density — their number per 1 mm^2 — also varies depending on the area. For instance, the melanocyte density is about 900 per mm^2 in the back and about 1500/mm^2 in the genital area (one of the most pigmented parts of the body). However, individual variations within the same body area are surprisingly small, even when comparing people of different races. Uniform distribution of melanocytes is preserved despite their different density in different body parts and is restored after their damage by UV radiation or due to other reasons (Thingnes J. et al., 2012).

Thus, the skin of people of different phototypes contains approximately the same number of melanocytes. Still, there are many nuances, primarily in the amount of melanin. People with dark skin have more melanin, the melanosomes are large and singly arranged, and the dendrites of the melanocytes are thicker and longer. In the skin of Caucasians and Asians, dendrites are thinner and shorter, there is less melanin, and melanosomes are mostly arranged in groups surrounded by a common shell, forming a so-called **melanosome complex** (**Fig. I-2-3**).

Moreover, in Asian skin, melanosomes are larger, packed more densely, and form more complexes than in Caucasian skin (**Fig. I-2-4**). It is assumed that the association of melanosomes in clusters helps to keep the smaller melanin granules of light skin from degradation longer (Zaidi K.U. et al., 2014; Hurbain I. et al., 2018).

Melanin distribution in keratinocytes also varies. In black

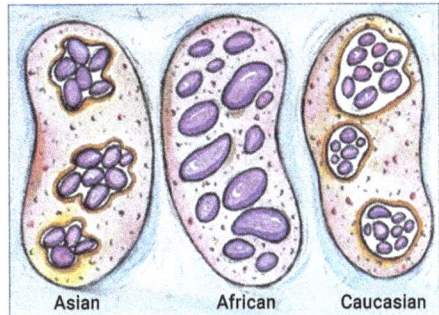

Figure I-2-3. Organization of melanin granules in the skin of racial groups

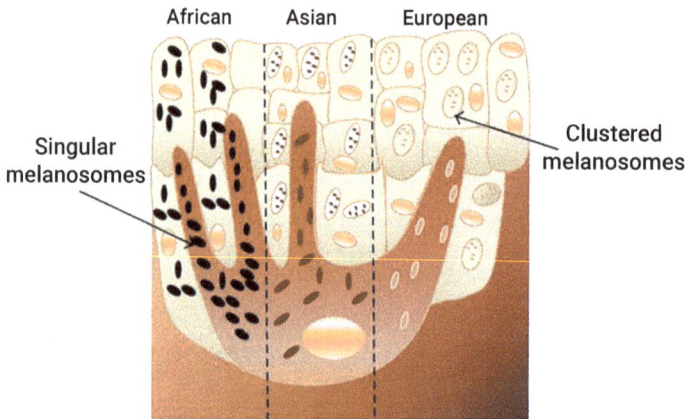

Figure I-2-4. Distribution of melanin granules and complexes in the skin of people of different races (adapted from Zaidi K.U. et al., 2014)

skin, melanin is evenly distributed throughout the epidermis from the basal layer to the *stratum corneum*. Melanin is also evenly distributed inside each keratinocyte — many large elliptical melanosomes reliably cover the cell nucleus. In Caucasoid skin, melanosomes are mainly concentrated in the basal layer and are destroyed inside keratinocytes long before they reach the uppermost layers of the epidermis (Visscher M.O., 2017). In contrast, the larger and more robust melanin granules of people with darker skin persist in the keratinocytes for quite a long time and are only released in the upper layers. Interestingly, according to Peter Elias, this may explain the more pronounced barrier properties of dark skin — perhaps the degradation products of melanosomes further acidify the epidermis of the upper layers. In addition, melanocytes of darker phototypes seem to send signals that stimulate the epidermis to produce more proteins, lipids, and enzymes, which is important for building a strong epidermal barrier (Elias P.M., 2005).

Moreover, although the amount of tyrosinase in different phototypes is similar, its activity is up to 10 times higher in dark phototypes than in people with phototype I (Valverde P. et al., 1995). Thus, people with dark skin are genetically programmed to continuously produce higher levels of melanin, even without UV exposure. We are talking specifically about eumelanin, which has photoprotective properties. As we said before, eumelanin and pheomelanin are always produced

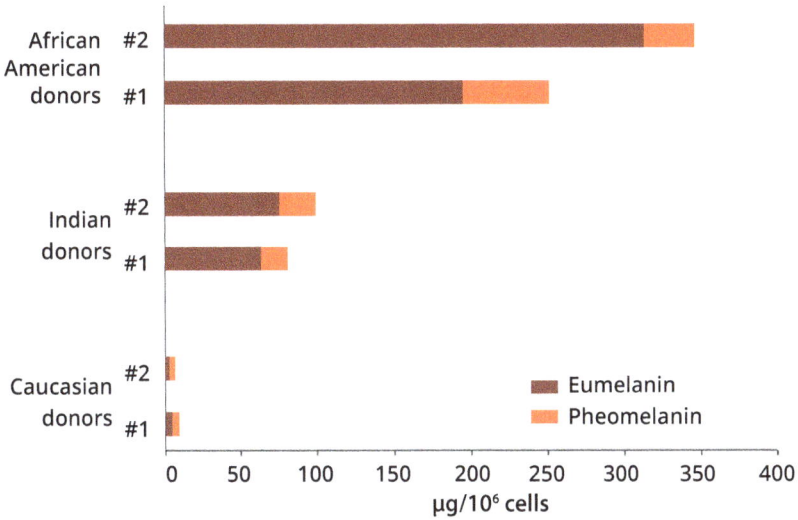

Figure I-2-5. Amount and eumelanin/pheomelanin ratio in the skin of individuals from different ethnic grroups (adapted from Kadekaro A.L. et al., 2006)

during melanogenesis. However, the higher the skin phototype, the more eumelanin is synthesized (**Fig. I-2-5**).

Red-haired people and people with fair skin have a very low amount of eumelanin. Most people with red hair and light skin have a dysfunctional variant of the MS1R receptor gene responsible for sensitivity to α-MSH and ACTH. Since the receptors do not work (or work poorly), the melanocytes of red-haired people respond poorly to hormonal stimuli and synthesize almost no eumelanin, only pheomelanin in the "background" mode. This accounts for the light coloring of the skin and red hair.

Unfortunately, as we mentioned above, pheomelanin not only has a poor protective ability against UV radiation compared to eumelanin but is also characterized by high phototoxicity and can enhance UV-induced ROS formation. Moreover, signaling pathways triggered by the activation of "healthy" receptor variants activate not only melanin synthesis but also antioxidant protection and acceleration of excision nucleotide repair. This helps in the fight against UV-induced DNA damage and prevents mutagenesis. In the case of defective MS1R polymorphisms found in Celtic phototypes, these mechanisms are also dysfunctional. Hence, they have a significantly increased risk

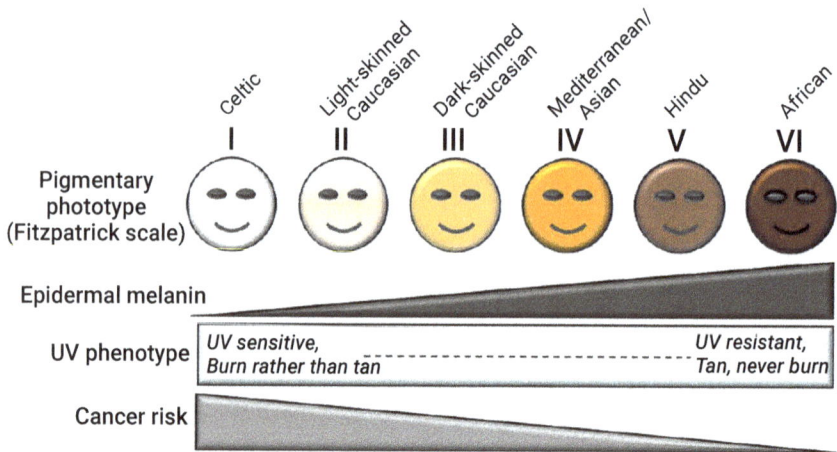

Figure I-2-6. Relationships between skin phototype, eumelanin content, and skin cancer risk (Image by Wikipedia.com)

of skin cancer and more pronounced signs of photoaging (**Fig. I-2-6**) (D'Orazio J. et al., 2013; Swope V.B., Abdel-Malek Z.A., 2018; Wolf Horrell E.M. et al., 2016).

The problem of defective MS1Rs is not unique to red-haired people (although they are homozygous, so the severity of the problems is greater). According to various data sources, up to 50% of Caucasoids are carriers of at least one copy of "weak" MS1R (heterozygous state) (Bauer J. et al., 2009). However, the second copy still compensates for the weak link — in people with phototype II, eumelanin content increases significantly, and pheomelanin level does not exceed 10%. In areas of constant sun exposure, even in fair-skinned people, the expression of tyrosinase and, to a greater extent, TYRP2, which turns colorless DHICA melanin into colored eumelanin, is increased. Presumably, the tyrosinase activity is changed, and therefore they begin to form a better tan with age (among other factors) (Alaluf S. et al., 2002; Alaluf S. et al., 2003).

As for people of Asian ethnicity, apart from the difference in melanin distribution in melanosomes, their melanocytes produce more eumelanin than those of Caucasoids. Generally, these people are more active and "responsive" to tanning. However, this is also the reason for their frequent development of melasma and post-inflammatory hyperpigmentation.

Chapter 3
Pigmentation-affecting factors

Pigmentation depends on internal and external factors.

Internal factors:
- Hereditary
- Endocrine disorders
- Inflammation
- Neurological disorders
- Nutrient deficiencies

External factors:
- Insolation
- Skin damage
- Exposure to chemicals
- Medications

3.1. Hormones, stress, and inflammation

3.1.1. Endocrine factors

Melanocytes contain not only receptors for α-MSH and ACTH but also estrogen receptors (cytosolic and nuclear), so they are sensitive to their change. Moreover, melanocytes of some people may be inherently more sensitive to the stimulating effects of estrogen and possibly to other sex steroid hormones, including progesterone (Jee S.H. et al., 1994). Hormone-induced melanogenesis can be associated with pregnancy and breastfeeding (increased α-MSH, estrogen, and progesterone production enhances the transcription of tyrosinase and DOPA-chromotomerase), menopause, taking oral hormonal contraceptives and hormone replacement drugs (in men, increasing testosterone), use of hormone-containing intrauterine devices (IUDs), thyroid and ovarian diseases, ACTH- and MSH-producing tumors, and Addison's disease.

3.1.2. Inflammation

Leukotrienes C4 and D4, prostaglandins E2 and D2, thromboxane-2, interleukins 1 and 6 (IL-1 and IL-6), tumor necrosis factor α (TNF-α), epidermal growth factor (EGF), and ROS (free radicals, nitric oxide) most actively affect melanogenesis during inflammation (Tomita Y. et al., 1992; Davis E.C., Callender V.D., 2010).

3.1.3. Stress

The hypothalamic–pituitary–adrenal system (HPA) is activated in response to stress factors. Thus, activation of releasing factors in the hypothalamus stimulates the secretion of ACTH, α-MSH, thyroid stimulating hormone (TSH), and human growth hormone (hGH) in the anterior pituitary lobe. The generated ACTH, in turn, stimulates the release of glucocorticosteroids (mainly cortisol), through which the main stress effects are realized. This system is called the central HPA axis.

The skin is not only influenced by processes occurring in the central axis of the HPA system; the skin itself responds directly to stress (**Fig. I-3-1**). In response to stress factors, epidermal keratinocytes, hair follicle keratinocytes, melanocytes, sebocytes, and mast cells produce the corticotropin-releasing hormone. Skin cells, including fibroblasts, can also produce ACTH and corticosterone. Neuropeptides (substance P) and neurotrophins released by free nerve endings and skin cells play a special role in neurogenic inflammation. These mechanisms together form the peripheral axis of the HPA system (Lin T.K. et al., 2017).

Together with the agents synthesized by the HPA, the substances formed directly in the skin cause a decrease in its barrier and immune function, activation of inflammatory processes, imbalance among free radicals, increased sebum production, disruption of epidermis proliferation and differentiation, delayed DNA reparation and damage healing, and stimulation of melanogenesis.

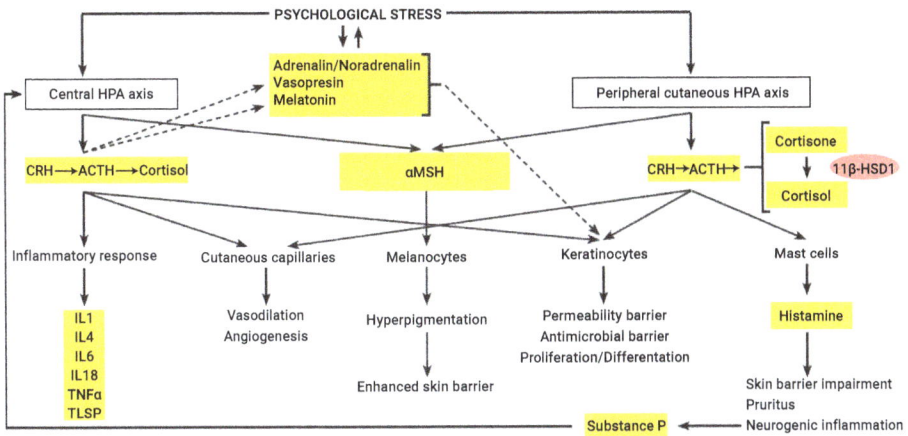

Figure I-3-1. The effect of psychological stress on the skin (adapted from Lin T.K. et al., 2017)

3.1.4. Nutrient deficiencies

There is no deficiency in the substrate for melanin synthesis. However, certain substances that influence the activity of melanogenesis enzymes or are involved in skin color formation may be deficient, such as vitamins B_1, B_2, C, B_5 (pantothenic acid), copper, iron, and zinc. The main dietary sources of these nutrients are listed in **Table I-3-1**.

Table I-3-1. Nutritional sources of vitamins and trace elements

NUTRIENT	FOOD
B_1	Yeast, bread, peas, cereals, walnuts, peanuts, liver, heart, egg yolk, milk, bran
B_2	Eggs, meat, liver, kidneys, fish, dairy products, cheese, broccoli, spinach, yeast
C	Fresh fruits, berries, vegetables, herbs, rosehips
B_5	Liver, kidneys, meat, heart, eggs, green vegetables, brewer's yeast, seeds, nuts
Cu	Hazelnuts, fresh cucumbers, avocados, rosehips
Fe	Meat, liver, kidneys, beans, hazelnuts, herbs
Zn	Oysters, mussels, cereals, veal liver, Brazil nuts

3.2. Solar radiation and tanning

Among the pigmentation-stimulating physical factors, the main place is occupied by UV radiation as one of the most aggressive environmental factors. Sun exposure plays a significant role in all types of pigmentation, which is why people living in warm climates are more often affected. They have a much larger skin area that is directly (and more intensely) exposed to the sun.

Today, UV exposure is recognized as the main culprit of premature skin aging. However, it is not only the danger of growing old early that should be of concern for sunbathers — UV rays can cause acute damage to the skin tissue, which is clinically manifested through burns, blisters, chronic inflammation, and pigment spots. In addition, UV light negatively affects the skin's immune function (e.g., it causes the conversion of the "protective" *trans*-urocanic acid into the *cis* form, which has an immunosuppressive effect and a direct and indirect damaging impact on immune cells). Yet, the most dangerous complication associated with the action of UV rays is malignant skin cell degeneration and the development of tumors. Skin can protect itself from UV light. The skin's natural "parasol" is the pigment melanin, although it turns out that it's not the only thing that provides photoprotection.

Skin is affected by both types of UV radiation reaching the Earth's surface — UVA and UVB (the ozone layer completely retains UVC):
- **UVB (280–320 nm)** is a harsher (more destructive) type of UV radiation, also known as tan UV. It is absorbed mainly in the epidermis and causes delayed pigmentation (after 3–7 days).
- **UVA (320–400 nm)** is milder radiation than UVB, capable of penetrating the dermis. It leads to immediate pigmentation, a phenomenon known as persistent skin darkening.

3.2.1. UV radiation

For light to have any effect on biological tissue (in this case, skin), it must be absorbed by it. The energy of absorbed light quanta is converted into other types of energy — thermal (then we feel the heat of sunlight) or chemical (then chemical reactions start to take place in the skin, which are usually either absent or very, very slow). The energy of UV radiation is mainly spent on photochemical transformations.

One way or another, ultraviolet light affects all skin cells — basal keratinocytes, mast cells, melanocytes, and blood vessel endothelial cells. This is partly due to the products of free radical reactions and the direct effect of UV radiation on the cells. In response to excess UV radiation, an adaptive response is triggered in the skin to reduce the dose of UV radiation reaching living cells. Specifically, the rate of division of basal keratinocytes increases, resulting in the thickening of the epidermis and the *stratum corneum* — an attempt to create a thick physical barrier to UV light. Melanocytes stimulate melanin synthesis, which not only acts as a solar "umbrella" and reduces the UV load on the skin in general, and keratinocytes in particular, but also influences the events unfolding in the skin after UV exposure. **Fig. I-3-2** provides a visual diagram of the reactions triggered in skin cells in response to

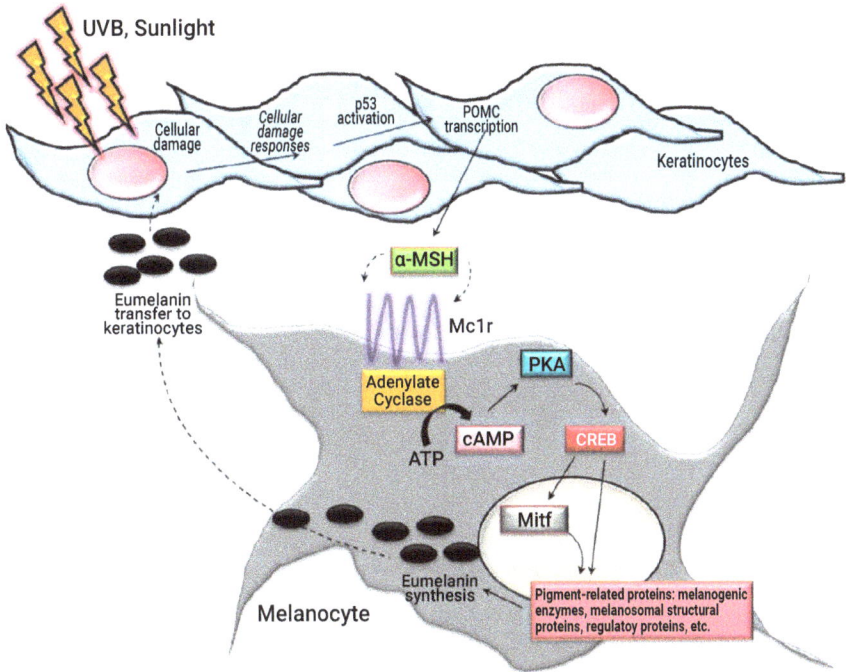

Figure I-3-2. Response of keratinocytes and melanocytes to UV light (adapted from D'Orazio J. et al., 2013)

UV light, and **Table I-3-2** shows the changes they lead to (Cichorek M. et al., 2013; D'Orazio J. et al., 2013).

Table I-3-2. Paracrine factors secreted by keratinocytes and dermal melanocytes after UV radiation and their effect on melanocyte biology (Cichorek M. et al., 2013)

SIGNAL MOLECULES	EFFECT ON MELANOCYTE
bFGF	↑ Proliferation
ET-1	↓ Proliferation ↑ Number and length of dendrites ↓ Melanogenesis
IL-1α/1β	↑ Proliferation ↑ Melanogenesis ↑ Cell survival rate
ACTH	↑ Proliferation ↑ Number and length of dendrites ↑ Melanogenesis ↑ Cell survival rate
α-MSG	↑ Number and length of dendrites ↑ Melanogenesis ↑ Melanosomal transfer
PGE2/PGEF2α	↑ Proliferation ↑ Melanogenesis
GM-CSF	↑ Melanogenesis
NO	↓ Melanogenesis
TNF-α	↑ Number and length of dendrites ↑ Cell survival rate
NGF	↓ Melanogenesis
BMP-4	↑ Proliferation ↑ Number and length of dendrites ↑ Melanogenesis

Abbreviations: bFGF — basic fibroblast growth factor; ET-1 — endothelin 1; IL — interleukin; ACTH — adrenocorticotropic hormone; α-MSH — melanocyte-stimulating hormone α; PGE2 — prostaglandin E2; PGF2α — prostaglandin F2α; GM-CSF — granulocyte-macrophage colony-stimulating factor; NO — nitric oxide; TNF-α — tumor necrosis factor α; NGF — nerve growth factor; BMP-4 — bone morphogenetic protein.

The mechanism of pigmentation formation in response to UV exposure — **tanning** — is primarily related to DNA damage:

- **Direct** in the case of UVB radiation — due to the direct absorption of photons in this energy range by DNA molecules and the formation of specific mutations, i.e., CPDs or pyrimidine-(6,4)-pyrimidine (6-4PP) photoproducts.
- **Indirect** in the case of UVA exposure. Under the influence of UVA radiation, ROS (superoxide anion, hydrogen peroxide, hydroxyl radical, singlet oxygen) are formed in the skin. Their interaction with DNA molecules leads to the formation of 8-oxo-2'-deoxyguanosine (8-oxo-dG, a marker of oxidative stress), single-stranded DNA breaks, and the formation of DNA-protein cross-links. In addition to DNA damage, ROS formed under the influence of UVA radiation also cause damage to other structures, e.g., proteins and fats (peroxidation of intercellular lipids and membrane lipids).

3.2.2. Tanning

Tanning is the body's adaptation to high seasonal levels of UV radiation, especially in the UVB range. Phenotypes with the capacity for tanning have evolved throughout human history, possibly due to independent mutations in genes controlling the pigmentation system and gene drift.

The formation of a tan involves two mechanisms:
1. Immediate pigment darkening (IPD)
2. Persistent pigment darkening (PPD)

Immediate pigment darkening (IPD)

IPD reaction involves an immediate skin darkening after UVA exposure with a maximum induction at 340 nm.

The effect produced by IPD is temporary. On light skin, it is immediately noticeable as irregular grayish–brown staining that occurs on areas that have been in contact with sunlight.

Cellular mechanisms of IPD are not fully understood, but they seem to involve both primarily photooxidation of colorless eumelanin precursors, DHICA and 6-hydroxy-5-methoxyindole-2-carboxylic acid

(6H5MICA), and spatial translocation of melanosomes within melanocytes and keratinocytes (Maeda K., Hatao M., 2004). In phenotypes with darker constitutive pigmentation, IPD develops faster and more intensively.

The cumulative effect of IPD is thought to be the immediate absorption or scattering of UV photons in the surface layers of the skin, thus preventing damage to the deeper layers. However, skin darkening from UVA exposure does not significantly increase melanin production or protect against sunburn, although it may persist for several weeks, taking on a brown tint.

Persistent pigment darkening (PPD)

PPD is usually considered tanning and is a process that leads to facultative pigmentation.

PPD develops gradually over a few hours, a few days, or possibly longer, depending on the duration of UVB radiation exposure (therefore, UVB is called tanning UV light). PPD involves melanin redistribution more toward the skin surface (as in the case of IPD), changes in the shape and intracellular arrangement of melanin (melanosomes accumulate around keratinocyte nuclei, forming a kind of shield), and, most importantly, promotes tyrosinase activation and synthesis of new eumelanin.

Since melanogenesis initiation takes time, this leads to a delayed appearance of tan, which is usually visible two or three days after exposure. This tan usually lasts for several weeks (in children, whose epidermal renewal rate is very high) or months (in adults) and even up to a year (in the elderly) — much longer than a tan caused by oxidation of existing melanin. This tanning mechanism protects the skin from UV radiation rather than simply serving a "cosmetic" function.

As a rule, the appearance of a tan provides additional protection equivalent to sun protection factor (SPF) 3 — meaning that tanned skin can withstand UV exposure until erythema (i.e., sunburn) forms three times longer than pale skin. However, it must be remembered that for it to start forming, it has to be preceded by photodamage to the DNA. That is, **a tan is a response to damage that may provide some degree of protection from subsequent UV exposure but not from its primary destructive effect**.

In addition to the tanning effect caused by acute sun exposure, delayed or long-term UV exposure leads to the appearance or aggravation of pigmented lesions.

3.3. Visible and infrared radiation

Recent research suggests that visible light can also cause pigmentation (Duteil L. et al., 2017).

The biological effects of human skin exposure to visible light were first described in 1962. In this work, the authors presented evidence that visible and long-wavelength UV radiation at physiological doses can cause pigmentation on human skin *in vivo* (Pathak M.A. et al., 1962a,b). However, compared to UV-induced hyperpigmentation, blue–violet light caused more pronounced darkening that persisted for up to three months, with molecular analysis showing decreased levels of p53 protein (regulates the cell cycle) (Mahmoud B.H. et al., 2010). Such a p53 response after exposure to blue−violet light suggests that the mechanisms of its effect on the skin are different from those involved in UVB action.

Recent studies have shown that opsin-3 receptors (OPN3) are activated in melanocytes under the influence of blue light, resulting in increased melanin synthesis. The authors of the first works on this subject associated this reaction with the induction of calcium current and kinase-dependent signaling cascade leading to microphthalmia-associated transcription factor (MITF) activation followed by increased expression of tyrosinase and dopachrome-tautomerase (Duteil L. et al., 2014).

However, in 2019, to confirm this hypothesis, a group of researchers from Brown University created a culture of melanocytes characterized by a reduced number of OPN3 on the cell membrane (Ozdeslik R.N. et al., 2019). It was assumed that the fewer OPN3 receptors, the less intracellular calcium levels would increase in response to irradiation, and therefore less intense pigmentation would be observed. However, when the scientists irradiated the cells with UV light, the amount of calcium in the cells still increased — just as it did in melanocytes with normal OPN3 quantities. Thus, OPN3 "didn't see" the UV light, just as they "didn't see" blue and green light. Moreover, the researchers established that the melanocytes with fewer OPN3 on their surface looked much darker because they had more melanin. That is, OPN3 did not increase but rather inhibited melanogenesis.

Subsequent experiments showed that in cells with a large amount of OPN3, the level of cAMP produced by MC1R decreased (Regazzetti C. et al., 2018). That is, the presence of OPN3 inhibited MC1R activity, preventing it from synthesizing too much cAMP. Consequently, it inhibited tyrosinase formation and subsequent melanin synthesis. Although the exact mechanisms of OPN3 functioning are still unclear (and these receptors are found in cells of other tissues as well), the discovery of its ability to regulate the amount of pigment in melanocytes allows considering it as a promising target for the treatment of various kinds of pigment disorders. It should be noted that the mechanisms of visible-light-induced hyperpigmentation do not involve ROS formation, so it is not eliminated by taking or topically applying antioxidants.

Despite previous assumptions, infrared (IR) light's ability to cause pigmentation has not been confirmed. Yes, the effect of near-IR light is indeed associated with increased expression of matrix metalloproteinases 1 and 9 (MMP-1 and MMP-9), degrading the collagen matrix and generating ROS. However, these levels of ROS do not lead to the formation of pigment lesions (Sondenheimer K., Krutmann J., 2018). Nonetheless, including antioxidants in sunscreen formulas can help protect dermal structures from IR light.

3.4. Air pollution

In recent years, the air pollution problem has received considerable attention, which is justified as it contributes significantly to the deterioration of human health. According to the World Health Organization (WHO), about eight million premature deaths annually are attributed to air pollution. Pollutants also affect the skin, with the main effects being the stimulation of pigmentation and premature skin aging. Let's briefly examine the primary pollutants and their contribution to pigmentation.

Particulate matter (PM) is an umbrella term for small solid or liquid particles suspended in the air:

- PM10 — 2.5–10 µm
- PM2.5 — 0.1–2.5 µm
- Ultrafine particles — less than 0.1 µm (< 100 nm)

The smaller the particles, the easier they penetrate the human body. Particles smaller than 1 µm can penetrate intact skin, and those of 2.4 µm diameter can enter the transfollicular route.

The main PM source is motor transport, as well as industrial emissions and dust from asphalted areas and unseeded soils.

In contact with skin, PM particles promote oxidative stress and inflammatory reactions, which leads to the degradation of the collagen framework and the formation of pigment spots. In addition, they can directly stimulate tyrosinase and enhance melanogenesis by acting on melanocyte aryl hydrocarbon receptors (AhR) (Peng F. et al., 2019). As a part of their study, Vierkötter A. et al. (2010) demonstrated that urban residents have 20% more pigment spots on the cheeks and 22% more on the forehead, as well as more pronounced nasolabial folds than rural residents, all other things being equal.

Nitrogen oxides (NO, NO_2) and sulfur oxides (SO_2) are oxidizing agents. Their main sources are fuel and energy complex enterprises, automobile transport, the chemical and oil refining industry, and the food industry. The damaging effect is associated with ROS formation and inflammation. An increase in the NO_2 concentration in the air by 10 µg/m^3 was associated with an increase in the number of pigment spots on the cheeks by 25% in Caucasian women and 24% in Chinese women (Hüls A. et al., 2016).

Polycyclic aromatic hydrocarbons (PAHs) are organic compounds formed during the combustion and processing of organic raw materials: oil products, coal, wood, garbage, food, and tobacco (the most famous representatives are benzanthracene, benzopyrene, anthracene, and naphthalene).

Tropospheric ozone is formed in cities under certain weather conditions and active operation of vehicles and industrial plants. These compounds also lead to the development of oxidative stress and inflammation, with PAHs directly stimulating AhR.

The aforementioned mechanisms are considered primary causes for the induction of pigment lesions by air pollutants (Parrado C. et al., 2019). Therefore, it should be said that **antioxidant and anti-inflammatory agents are currently the main anti-pollution agents**.

Chapter 4
Evolution of pigmentation: adaptation to UV radiation

Concluding our story on the pigmentation biology and physiology, we would like to explain why people have different skin colors — how pigmentation arose in the first place and for what purpose. Scientists have long considered skin color as an evolutionary "response" of the human body to living under conditions characterized by varying intensity of UV exposure. Renowned American anthropologist Nina Jablonski and her colleague George Chaplin substantiated this assumption and linked it to the reproductive function necessary to preserve the human species (Jablonski N.G., Chaplin G., 2010a,b).

As we know, our skin needs UV light to synthesize vitamin D_3, which is necessary for calcium absorption and normal growth. However, too high a UV dose can deplete other vital substances in the body and cause malignant changes in skin cells. Melanin, the skin pigment, works as a natural "parasol," absorbing UV rays as soon as they enter the skin. The darker the skin, the stronger the protection.

Jablonski and Chaplin calculated the dose of UV radiation people living at different latitudes need for normal vitamin D_3 production (**Fig. I-4-1**). Then, they compared their calculations with a map of the distribution of UV levels on the Earth's surface, compiled from National Aeronautics and Space Administration (NASA) satellite data (Del Bino S. et al., 2018).

They found that the skin can be very dark in the equatorial zone and still produce enough vitamin D_3. However, in more northern latitudes, the skin must lighten to absorb the necessary amount of UV light. Otherwise, the body becomes deficient in this vitamin due to decreased synthesis. Indeed, the skin of people native to equatorial regions is the darkest. But its tone gets lighter as you move away from the equator.

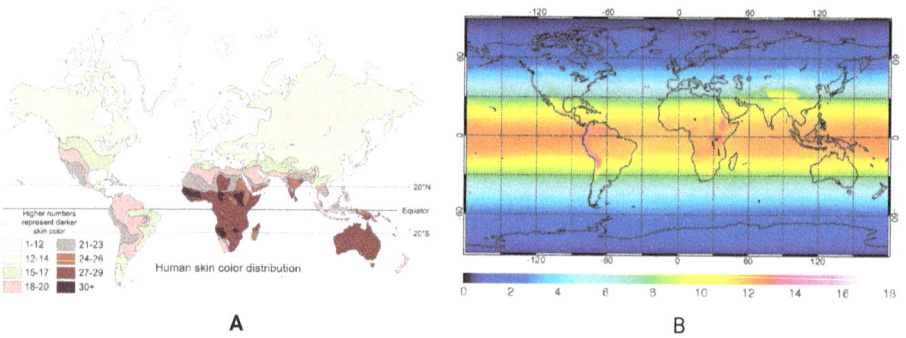

Figure I-4-1. Map of human skin color distribution (A) and UV levels at the Earth's surface (B) (Image by Wikipedia.com)

UV radiation has another important effect: it promotes the photolysis of folate, a key nutrient for embryonic development and sperm production. Thus, scientists believe that **skin color is a kind of compromise betweentwo different "levers" acted on by UV. On the one hand, the skin must be light enough to allow the necessary dose of UV for vitamin D$_3$ synthesis. On the other hand, it must be dark enough to protect folate from destruction and thereby ensure the normal functioning of the reproductive system**.

4.1. Internal "levers of pressure" in the evolution of pigmentation

After establishing that UV radiation does not simply correlate with but is the cause of variability in human skin pigmentation, work began to identify possible selection mechanisms.

4.1.1. Why sunburn, cancer, and vitamin D overproduction are not evolutionary "levers" of pigmentation

For most of the twentieth century, the debate over the value of dark pigmentation for selection focused on the protective effects of melanin against burns, skin cancer, and overproduction of vitamin D.

However, these factors cannot be considered significant components of selection pressure. Sunburn and skin cancer have negligible effects on reproductive success.

Skin cancer, except for melanoma, is common among older people from light-skinned populations who live in areas with high levels of sun exposure, but it rarely results in death or incapacitation. Melanoma is often fatal in younger people, but it is much less common than other skin cancers.

Still, when considering the evolutionary significance of skin cancer, current statistics on its prevalence need to be examined carefully. The highest prevalence of skin cancer is found in people with light pigmentation who are exposed to intense episodic or regular heavy UV exposure in areas far from their ancestral homelands. **Skin cancer is most often the result of modern human migration, i.e., the outcome of a mismatch between skin pigmentation and the geographic area or lifestyle.**

Skin cancer now has a moderate effect on human reproductive success, and it may have been statistically insignificant when humans could not yet move quickly and migrate across long distances. Genetic data indicating no significant association between 15 single-nucleotide polymorphisms (**Fig. I-4-2**) and the risk of developing skin cancer further confirm this assumption.

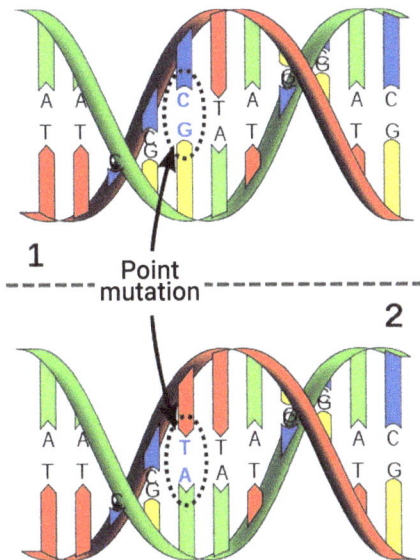

Figure I-4-2. A single-nucleotide polymorphism is a nucleotide substitution in a single nucleotide pair of DNA. It results from point mutations (https://www.wikidoc.org/index.php/ Single_nucleotide_polymorphism)

Overproduction of vitamin D as the main cause of dark pigmentation evolution was rejected after it was discovered that the development of hypervitaminosis D from sun exposure is physiologically impossible due to photochemical regulation.

Since the traditionally considered factors in the evolution of skin pigmentation proved inconclusive, we revised the possible acting forces of selection.

4.1.2. Folate is the key

The assumption that photolysis of folate under the influence of sunlight could be a determining factor in the evolution of dark pigmentation was first suggested before the role of folate in biosynthesis, repair, DNA methylation, amino acid metabolism, and melanin production was fully understood.

Jablonski and Chaplin further refined the theory that dark skin in humans evolved primarily because of the need to prevent decreased fertility due to the photolysis of folate in skin vessels. They presented evidence that depletion of folate by UV exposure would lead to folate deficiency in the body, which in turn would cause the development of potentially fatal congenital abnormalities such as neural tube defects (NTDs) — the most common birth defects in humans.

Further studies on folate photosensitivity under various *in vitro* and *in vivo* conditions have shown that **there is a complex relationship between skin pigmentation and folate metabolism, involving both direct photodegradation of folate (in its basic form 5-methyltetrahydrofolate, 5-MTHF) and its photodegradation in the presence of flavins and porphyrins under the influence of reactive oxygen species (ROS)**. Serious epidemiological studies are needed to investigate the relationship among skin pigmentation, folate metabolism, and NTD prevalence. However, the protective effect of dark pigmentation, which prevents folate depletion and NTDs, is evident.

Folate is particularly important for the rapidly dividing germ and seminal tubule cells. Thus, folate deficiency caused by intense UV radiation could affect both male and female fertility. Low folate levels cause folate-mediated one-carbon metabolism disorders, which can lead to severe diseases and malformations. Folate deficiency causes defective DNA replication due to strand breaks stemming from errors in incorporating excess uracil into DNA. Maintaining adequate folate levels results in a 72% reduction in NTD incidence. This is due to the direct effect of folate in normalizing neural tube development owing to the role it plays in the division of rapidly dividing cells. Folate deficiency also disrupts nucleotide excision repair, the main mechanism for removing UV-derived photoproduced DNA.

The maintenance of folate metabolism is of high evolutionary importance because it directly affects reproductive success and early life survival. Due to the multifaceted involvement of folate and its derivatives in cell division, DNA repair, and melanin production, and the fact that these substances are degraded by UV radiation and ROS, intensive natural selection has taken place to protect normal folate levels.

Competition for folate can be intense, especially when the body is stressed by UV exposure and a lack of folate in the diet. Recent studies have shown that folate regulates melanin production because it is required for synthesizing guanosine triphosphate (GTP), a substrate for *de novo* production of tetrahydrobiopterin (BH4) and 6BH4 in melanocytes and keratinocytes. In turn, 6BH4 regulates tyrosinase activity in melanosomes.

4.1.3. Vitamin D is the next candidate for the internal "lever" of natural selection

The evolution of light pigmentation at high latitudes has long been attributed to the importance of vitamin D production in the skin under insufficient sunlight. Vitamin D_3 synthesis begins in the skin when 7-dehydrocholesterol (7-DHC) absorbs UV radiation, resulting in the formation of pre-vitamin D_3. This reaction occurs only under the influence of UVB radiation in the 290–310 nm wavelength range, with maximum transformation at 295–297 nm. The photosynthesis of vitamin D_3 in the skin depends on the sun's zenith angle, which varies with the season, geographic latitude, and time of day. It is also controlled by the amount of pigment and skin thickness.

The importance of vitamin D_3 as a selection driver in the skin pigmentation evolution is related to the multiple health effects of this vitamin.

Vitamin D_3 is involved in the regulation of many independent biological processes, including bone metabolism, innate immune response, and cell proliferation and differentiation. The role of vitamin D_3 in intestinal calcium absorption regulation and bone formation and remodeling has been known for decades. The important role of vitamin D_3 in establishing and maintaining innate immunity and the normal functioning of the pancreas, brain, and heart was relatively recently established. Reduced fertility due to vitamin D_3 deficiency is most pronounced in alimentary rickets. However, it is also significantly associated with an increased incidence of bacterial and viral infections and the risk of autoimmune diseases such as multiple sclerosis and type I diabetes.

Natural selection to ensure continuous production of vitamin D in the body by reducing pigmentation in populations living in areas with lower UV exposure was very strong. Such a selection was hypothesized even before the genetic evidence was available. Genetic verification of three independent evolutionary pathways of depigmented skin in hominin populations was noted in lineages leading to modern inhabitants of Northern Europe and East Asia, as well as in *Homo neanderthalensis*. It is a curious fact that the genetic and physiological mechanisms causing the formation of light-skinned phenotypes in each group were different (Jablonski N.G., Chaplin G., 2010a,b).

Regulatory mechanisms include control of melanosome formation and production of different types and combinations of melanin. Recently, the mechanisms by which different genetic pathways achieved the same phenotypic results have been addressed (Lucock M.D., 2022). One of the most interesting questions of vitamin D physiology in humans yet to be answered concerns the nature of variation in vitamin D receptors and especially whether their structure polymorphism is related to UVB levels and/or duration of exposure to certain UVB conditions.

4.2. External force of natural selection: UV radiation

A growing body of evidence demonstrating the role of natural selection in the formation and maintenance of phenotypes with dark or light skin pigmentation in areas close to the equator or the poles, re-spectively, has prompted scientists to look more closely at the nature of the external acting force of selection — UV radiation.

4.2.1. Geographic variations of UV radiation

Differences in the intensity, seasonal distribution, and biological activity of UVA and UVB radiation have long been known. However, their contribution to the evolution of human skin pigmentation has been underestimated. Hominin migrations from the African continent, which occurred about 1.9 million years ago and 80,000 years ago, were accompanied by the movement of humans from areas with high levels of UV radiation to places with much more heterogeneous UV exposure, characterized by seasonal variations, different intensity, and spectral combinations. Although two separate branches of hominins (early *Homo* and *Homo sapiens*, respectively) participated in these dispersals, neither of them made or used clothing or other portable means of protection against solar radiation. Thus, except for the time they spent in the shade, their bodies were fully exposed to UV radiation.

The fraction of UVA rays reaching the Earth's surface is higher than the fraction of UVB rays because UVB radiation is scattered and ab-sorbed by oxygen, ozone, and water molecules in the atmosphere. Due to this circumstance and the "geometry" (i.e., the angle of incidence) of sunlight in different places and in different seasons, the intensity and distribution of UVB radiation exhibit much greater variability than those of UVA.

UVB levels are highest in areas near the equator, drier areas, and at higher elevations, such as the Tibetan Plateau and the Altiplano Plateau (**Fig. I-4-3A**). At about 46° north and south, UVB levels are in-sufficient for most of the year to initiate provitamin D_3 production in the skin. Geographic latitude has the greatest influence on the pat-tern of UVB distribution due to the scattering and absorption of rays in the atmosphere. Africa is characterized by uniform and high levels of UVB radiation, while in northern Eurasia, its levels are very low. The coefficient of variation (CV) for UVB (**Fig. I-4-3B**) has a strong relationship with off-tropical seasonality. It is lowest at the equator and highest in northern Eurasia and North America. Humidity and

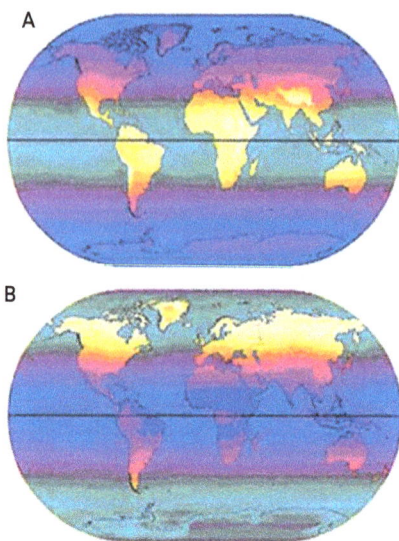

Figure I-4-3. A — annual mean UVB (305 nm) levels. Intensities are shown as gradations in ten degrees from dark to light, ranging from 1 to 135 J/m^2, with the oceans partially colored in gray; B — one-year coefficient of variation for UVB (305 nm) intensity. Ten-degree gradations from dark to light range from 10 to 300, with oceans partially colored in gray (adapted from Jablonski N.G., Chaplin G., 2010a)

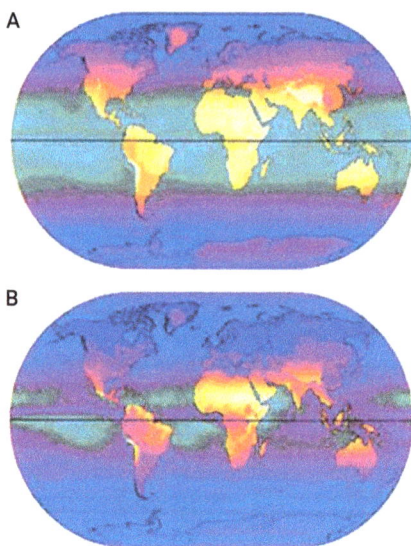

Figure I-4-4. A — annual mean UVA (380 nm) levels. Intensities are shown as gradations in ten degrees from dark to light, ranging from 65 to 930 J/m^2, with the oceans partially colored in gray; B — one-year coefficient of variation for UVA (380 nm) intensity. Gradations from dark to light in ten degrees ranging from 1 to 13, with the oceans partially colored in gray (adapted from Jablonski N.G., Chaplin G., 2010a)

monsoon precipitation contribute to the decrease in mean UVB levels, and CV has a more significant relationship with mean levels in areas with high humidity.

UVA radiation is observed closer to the poles (**Fig. I-4-4A**). UVA intensity at 380 nm is about 15 times greater than UVB at 305 nm, with an average UVA intensity of 283–570 J/m^2 in Western Europe compared to 20–40 J/m^2 for UVB. UVA intensity is slightly lower in regions close to the equator than in tropical and subtropical regions. The reflectivity of light-colored soil and especially snow contributes to higher UVA levels; atmospheric humidity does not affect levels in other regions. The CV for the annual UVA levels (**Fig. I-4-4B**) is almost the reverse of that of UVB, and is approximately 1/200 of the CV in UVB radiation. UVA intensity varies mostly in the dry tropical regions and has low levels of variation away from the equator.

To summarize, comparing UVB patterns at the equator and in the tropics with those outside tropical regions is reasonable. The average UVB values are high at the equator and in the tropics, with two seasonal peaks at equinoxes. Average UVA levels at the equator and in the tropics are also very high but have more variation in intensity throughout the year. Outside the tropics, average UVB levels are much lower and have a single peak during the summer solstice. Low average UVB levels in northern Eurasia and North America correspond to high CV. Note that there are no comparable populated land masses in the Southern Hemisphere with low UVB levels except for the southern tip of South America. Average UVA levels outside the tropics are lower, but they also exhibit less variation. This indicates that UVB levels at these latitudes are lower but more stable throughout the year.

Solar radiation was constantly changing in a timeframe limited by the lifespan and dispersal of hominins. Solar radiation and insolation are not static; they change according to different time cycles and over time. Insolation depends on the degree and features of the Sun's magnetic field lines on or near its surface. Shorter-wavelength insolation varies mainly due to energy changes in the flocculus and flare network on the Sun. UVB levels can vary by minutes and days and according to solar rotation cycles (27 days) and the 11-year sunspot cycle; longer-period fluctuations occur every few decades and centuries. The total solar irradiance varies only within 0.1–0.3%, but the variability of the short-wave UV spectrum can be an order of magnitude higher. For example, it has been found that during the Little Ice Age (1500–1800 AD), UV radiation levels were 4–10 times lower than they are today. Orbital parameters change the insolation pattern according to Milankovitch cycles every 22,000 years.

Currently, the Southern Hemisphere has higher extremes with intense insolation in summer, while the Northern Hemisphere has lower extremes and more insolation in winter. Nevertheless, the average annual insolation values in the land masses in the Southern and Northern hemispheres are unequal. In addition, the distribution of land masses between the two hemispheres is such that most of the Southern Hemisphere is characterized by high levels of UV radiation, while most of the Northern Hemisphere is characterized by extremely low levels.

4.2.2. UV as a driving force of selection in the pigmentation evolution

UV radiation has been a powerful creative force in the evolution of life on Earth, and organisms have developed several defenses against its specific wavelengths.

As previously argued, bare skin was the primary boundary between the human body and solar radiation for most of the history of the genus Homo. In equatorial Africa, members of the genus of early *Homo* and later *Homo sapiens* were exposed to the powerful "mix" of UVA and UVB radiation that prevailed in the tropics throughout the year. UVA radiation can penetrate deep into the skin and reach the dermal layer. UVB has more energy, but because it is absorbed and scattered in the upper layers of the epidermis, it does not reach the dermal layer.

In geographic areas with high UV levels, the human skin and body (**Table I-4-1**) were subjected to strong pressures of natural selection, leading to permanent dark constitutive pigmentation and the ability to increase eumelanin levels in response to seasonal increases in UVB levels. This adaptive trait was fixed genetically by eliminating the polymorphism at the MC1R locus.

When humans dispersed from the tropics to South Africa and from Africa to the rest of the Earth, they entered regions with low average annual UV levels and vastly different seasonal "proportions" of UVA and UVB radiation. Outside of the tropics, humans encountered two major changes in the UV regime.

1. The first was a transition from high annual UVB levels with two intensity peaks at equinoxes to relatively low annual UVB levels with one annual peak at the summer solstice.
2. The second was a dramatic decrease in the duration and intensity of UVB exposure as geographic latitude increased by every degree, so that most of the Northern Hemisphere remained

Table I-4-1. Effects of UVA and UVB radiation on the human body and the selection mechanisms involved in the evolution of pigmentation

SUGGESTED MECHANISMS	IMPACT
UVA radiation	
Photolysis of folate — in the form of 5-methyltetrahydrofolate (5-MTHF) —directly and via ROS in the presence of flavins and porphyrins, leading to a reduction in folate required for cell division	+++
Competition for folate: the increased need for folate for DNA repair and methylation processes, where it acts as a single-carbon donor, competes with the folate requirements for melanogenesis processes	++
Impaired melanin production due to tyrosinase sensitivity to high ROS level	++
Malignant melanoma (the only skin cancer that causes death in people of reproductive age)	+
Photoconversion of excess vitamin D_3 into inactive metabolites	+
Production of pyrimidine cyclobutane dimers and nucleotide damage resulting from photon absorption by DNA, requiring repair; activation of folate-mediated DNA repair processes	+++
Direct photolysis of folate (in the form of 5-MTHF in serum), resulting in a reduction in the amount of folate available for cell division processes and regulation of tyrosinase activity during melanogenesis	+
UVB radiation	
Competition for folate: the increased need for folate for DNA repair processes and for DNA methylation processes, where it acts as a single-carbon donor, competes with the folate requirements for melanogenesis processes	+
Sunburn	–
Damage to DNA and its repair system and disorders of the immune system, leading to the progression of genetic damage and the formation of non-melanocytic skin cancers	–
Dermal photosynthesis of vitamin D_3	–
The greater need for vitamin D in women may have caused an increase in sexual dimorphism in pigmentation, enhanced by the action of sexual selection in some populations	–

"+" — selection pressure to skin pigmentation; "–" — no effect.

without UVB energy for more than six months of the year. (The only exception to this rule was and is the Tibetan Plateau, which, due to its enormous altitude and thinning atmosphere, has significantly higher annual and summer UVB levels than other areas at the same latitude.)

Reduced UVB levels and, consequently, the potential for dermal biosynthesis of vitamin D created a positive selection that promoted depigmentation. Hominins and modern humans independently migrated beyond tropical latitudes, and depigmented phenotypes evolved in them through myriad pathways with a genetic basis, some of which have yet to be established. It is important to emphasize that living in middle latitudes — roughly between 23° and 46° — caused the evolution of partially depigmented phenotypes capable of tanning.

4.2.3. UV radiation and the evolution of the skin's ability to tan

From an evolutionary perspective, the importance of the delayed tan formation we discussed above is that it does not occur immediately, and the "base tan" develops slowly. Outside tropical latitudes, a slow rise in UVB amounts in spring to the levels capable of inducing provitamin D_3 photosynthesis provides good conditions for vitamin D_3 production and storage before facultative pigmentation develops in the skin because of ROS competition for UVB photons. Under slowly increasing UVB levels, skin burns would be rare and would not pose a potential threat to survival or reproductive success.

People spent a considerable amount of time outdoors without clothes and were exposed to gradual changes in UV intensity and combinations of wavelengths in different seasons. They didn't go far from home to vacation in sunnier areas and didn't use tanning beds. Modern doctors consider the ability to tan to be a suboptimal way to adapt to UV radiation because it causes damage to the connective tissue in the skin, the immune system, and DNA and thus leads to progressive changes that may lead to the development of skin cancer. This statement is true for free-living, long-lived people of the 21st century but not for those who lived in the 18th century or earlier, before the invention of widely available fast ways to travel long distances. In early humans and before increased life expectancy due to improved nutrition and medical advances, skin cancer did not affect reproductive success. Furthermore, the genetic pattern of skin cancer risk is inconsistent with predictions based on selection to resist skin cancer. So, in the context of human evolution, the development of the ability to form a tan was truly a perfect evolutionary compromise.

4.3. Conclusion

The visual representation of UVA and UVB levels and variations allows us to study the selection mechanisms involved in the evolution of differences in skin pigmentation and especially the evolution of phenotypes with the ability to form a tan under seasonal changes in UVB levels. Skin pigmentation is probably one of the best examples of the influence of natural selection on the formation of traits in humans. It is the product of two opposing clines*.

One promoted dark constitutive pigmentation and photoprotection from high UVA and UVB levels near the equator (see **Fig. I-4-3** and **I-4-4**). The other led to the development of light constitutive pigmentation to ensure the continuity of seasonal, UVB-induced photosynthesis of vitamin D_3 in areas close to the poles. At intermediate latitudes with seasonal fluctuations in UVB levels, the evolutionary conditions for humans with medium constitutive pigmentation and the ability to tan have developed.

As hominins settled outside the tropics, they encountered different intensities and seasonal combinations of UVA and UVB radiation. High UVA doses prevailed throughout the year in the tropics, with two equinox peaks in the UVB amount. Under these conditions, the main selection pressure was to protect folate by maintaining dark pigmentation. Photolysis of folate and its major serum form 5-methylhydrofolate occurs under the influence of UV light as well as ROS generated by UVA radiation. Under high UV stress conditions, there is strong competition

---

* Clinal variability (cline) is a continuous, gradual change in a trait throughout a species' range or in part of its range. It results from populations' adaptation to gradations of abiotic or biotic environmental factors.

for folate among the processes of cell division, DNA repair, and melanogenesis, exacerbated by inadequate nutrition. Outside tropical latitudes, low UVB levels are mainly observed, with only one peak per year. Populations with the most depigmented skin inhabit areas with the lowest annual levels and summer peaks of UVB.

The development of facultative pigmentation (tanning) was essential for populations inhabiting latitudes in the 23° to 46° approximate range, where UVB levels exhibit significant seasonal variations. Depigmented skin and skin capable of tanning have varied countless times during hominid evolution through independent genetic pathways under the influence of positive selection.

The almost complete absence in African populations of functionally significant variations in the coding region of the melanocortin-1 receptor (MC1R), one of the major genes regulating eumelanin production in humans, points to the action of purifying selection to maintain dark pigmentation under intense natural selection pressure. It is now thought that the persistence of MC1R in light-skinned individuals is not due to positive selection for this gene but because the lack of high irradiation in Northern Europe has weakened the pressure of natural selection on MC1R activity, allowing the gene that encodes it to mutate into a dysfunctional variant (Del Bino S. et al., 2018).

Evidence of functional restriction of MC1R in African populations is infrequent, given the high levels of polymorphism observed in other DNA loci in these populations.

There is growing evidence that dark-pigmented skin or the facultative ability to develop dark pigmentation when tanning evolved secondarily to positive selection in populations migrating from low to high UV regions. Changes in pigmentation such as these appear to have occurred after the migration of light and medium-pigmented "northern Indian ancestors" to the far reaches of the Indian Peninsula with high UV levels and in East Asians with light and medium pigmentation during their migration to the Central and mountainous areas of South America with high UV levels. Further studies of the genomic evidence for selecting genes responsible for pigmentation in human populations are needed to prove this claim.

The change in pigmentation over the course of an individual's life reflects its importance to reproduction and, consequently, to the evolution of the human species. Children are born with lighter pigmentation than adults, and their constitutive pigmentation develops to a genetically determined maximum only by the end of the second or the beginning of the third decade when they reach the period of maximum fertility. The maximum potential for the development of facultative pigmentation also occurs during maturity. In middle-aged and older people, constitutive pigmentation decreases, and the potential for tanning decreases due to a decline in the number of active melanocytes.

Skin pigmentation is an attractive model system for understanding and studying evolution. It is easy to see, and the basic mechanisms contributing to its development are easy to understand. Skin pigmentation meets the criteria for a successful evolutionary model:

- First, a non-ideal replicator gene is responsible for its development. Pigmentation is determined by germline DNA subject to mutation. Pigmentation also depends on inherited variations in epigenetic transmission due to DNA methylation, as well as on sexual partner preference associated with different cultural traditions.
- Second, selection should occur through differences in the survival rates of different phenotypes. In the case of skin pigmentation, this implies differences in the survival and reproductive rates of different phenotypes under different insolation conditions.
- Third, natural selection must be separated in time and space to understand the development of isolating mechanisms. In the evolution of skin pigmentation, isolation was caused by distance and human dispersal rather than by sexual selection or other mechanisms.

Thus, human skin is an ideal model for demonstrating the mechanisms of evolution by natural selection on all necessary parameters.

Part II

Clinical picture & pigmentation analysis

Human skin color contrast, determined by the content and distribution of concentrations of melanin and hemoglobin chromophores, plays a major role in the perception of age, health, and attractiveness.

Pigmentation disorders — **dyschromias** — are the third most common skin problem. Their peculiarity is the absence of any complaints and deterioration of health, but a significant impact on patients' quality of life.

1.1. Pigmentation disorders

All types of pigmentary disorders are divided into two large groups: **hyperpigmentations** associated with excessive accumulation of melanin in the epidermis and/or dermal layer and **hypopigmentations** caused by a reduction or absence of melanin. The latter is less common and very difficult to treat. Most often, specialists deal with hyperpigmentations. The good news is that we have many ways to treat them.

Several classifications of pigmentary disorders are used in clinical practice.

According to the **pigment distribution** in the skin layers:
1. Superficial — melanin is mostly accumulated in the epidermis
2. Deep — the pigment is found both in epidermis and dermis

Clinical types of pigmentation disorders differ in the depth of excess melanin:
1. Epidermal:
   - Freckles
   - Lentigo simple, sunny
   - Seborrheic keratosis

- Speckled nevus
- Café-au-lait spots
- Epidermal melasma

2. Dermo-epidermal (mixed):
   - Congenital melanocytic nevi
   - Acquired melanocytic nevi
   - Post-inflammatory hyperpigmentation
   - Becker's nevus
   - Mixed melasma

3. Dermal:
   - Nevus of Ota (ocular dermal melanosis)
   - Nevus of Ito (looks like nevus of Ota, but localized in the neck and upper torso)
   - Mongolian spot (a pathology of patients of the African and Mongoloid races; in persons with fair skin, it occurs in only 1–10% of cases);
   - Dermal melasma

According to the **origin**:
- Pigmentary disorders associated with hereditary diseases (e.g., black acanthosis, neurofibromatosis, Peitz–Jeghers disease, pigment incontinence)
- Skin malformations and neoplasms (melanocytic nevi, DuBray's melanosis, melanoma, lentigo)
- Hormonal influences (melasma in pregnant women, Addison's disease, acromegaly, hypothyroidism)

According to the **pathogenesis**, the following pigmentary disorders are distinguished:
- Associated with an increase in the number of melanocytes
- Associated with an increase in melanin
- Non-melanin disorders

1.1.1. Pigmentation disorders associated with an increase in the number of melanocytes

These are pigmented nevi, lentigo, Peitz–Jeghers–Touraine syndrome, Mongolian spot, nevus of Ota, and nevus of Ito.

Pigmented nevi

Pigmented nevi are light to dark brown spots or plaques that usually appear at birth or in the early years of life. Their surface is smooth or bumpy and may be covered with hairs. Pigmented nevi gradually grow, ranging in diameter from 0.5 cm to several centimeters.

Lentigo

A lentigo is a yellowish to dark brown pigmented spot. There are two varieties: solar and senile.

Sun lentigines are small brown spots of varying sizes that resemble moles and are located on areas of skin exposed to the sun — the face, upper back, shoulders, and back of the hands (**Fig. II-1** and **II-2**). Solar lentigo is considered a sign of photoaging. The keratinocyte growth factor, produced by fibroblasts and stimulating melanogenesis, is important in solar lentigo (Hasegawa K. et al., 2015).

Senile lentigines are more common in older women. Still, they may appear much earlier (from age 30) and are represented by single large spots 1–2 cm in diameter with clear boundaries of uniform light or dark brown color, located mainly on the face (**Fig. II-3**).

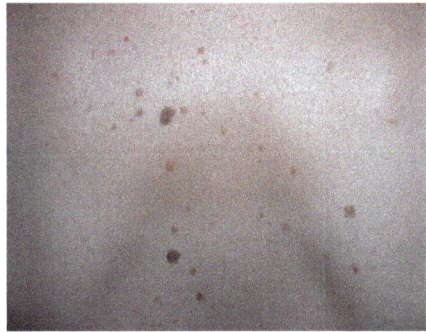

Figure II-1. Solar lentigo on the back (Image by Albanova V.I.)

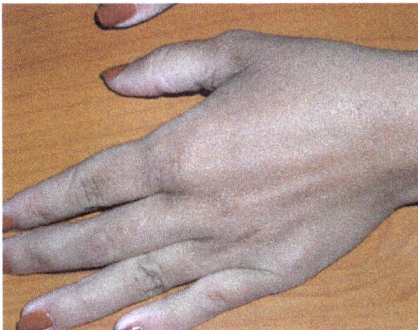

Figure II-2. Solar lentigo on the hand (Image by Albanova V.I.)

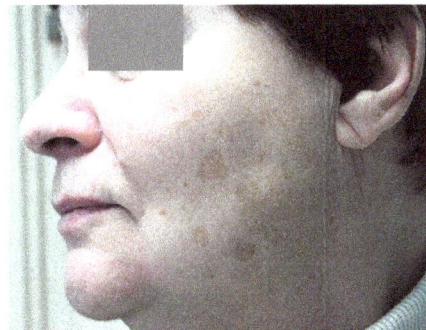

Figure II-3. Age spots on the face (Image by Albanova V.I.)

Peitz–Jeghers–Touraine syndrome

Multiple pigment spots are called lentiginosis. A special variant is a periorificial lentiginosis or Peitz–Jeghers–Touraine syndrome. It is a hereditary disease in which small brown or black, rounded spots are located periorificially, invading the mucosa of the mouth, mainly the lower lip. The spots are combined with polyposis of the gastrointestinal tract.

Mongolian spot

It is a large rounded or oval bluish pigmentation lesion of without sharp boundaries, noticeable at birth in the sacral region (mostly affecting Asians). The spot subsides by the age of 1–2 years.

Nevus of Ota

Nevus of Ota (oculodermal melanosis) is a deep dermal pigmentation located along the I and II branches of the trigeminal nerve, often unilateral. Blue–gray spots of varying sizes can evolve, besides the skin, the mucous membranes of the eye, nose, and pharynx. Nevus of Ota occurs predominantly in women and belongs to the melanoma-risky pigmented nevi.

Nevus of Ito

Nevus of Ito is clinically similar to nevus of Ota. However, the pigmentation is located on the skin areas innervated by the lateral branches of the supraclavicular nerve and the lateral cutaneous nerve of the shoulder, on the skin of the neck, above the clavicle, on the scapula, or in the deltoid muscle. This type of nevus is also a precancerous lesion. The histological picture of both nevi corresponds to intradermal nevus.

1.1.2. Pigmentation disorders associated with an increase in melanin

Increased melanin is associated with café-au-lait spots, freckles, melasma (chloasma), post-inflammatory pigmentation, pigmentation due to skin diseases, and drug-induced lesions.

Café-au-lait spots

Large and small homogeneously colored, well-defined, evenly bordered, café-au-lait spots occur mainly in neurofibromatosis but also in some syndromes (e.g., Mc-Queen–Albright, Hunter, Bloom, Cowden, Fanconi, Louis–Barr, LEOPARD, Maffucci) and appear in childhood (**Fig. II-4**).

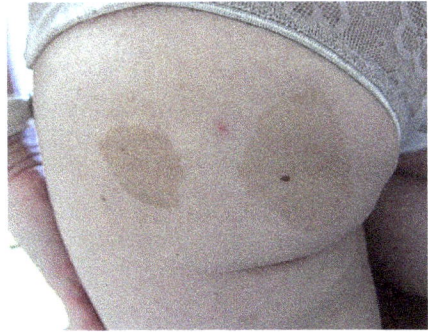

Figure II-4. Large café-au-lait spots on the buttock of a patient with neurofibromatosis (Image by Albanova V.I.)

Freckles

Freckles (ephelides) are a genetically determined seasonal pigmentation of exposed body areas. It appears in individuals of both sexes with phototypes I and II from 4–6 to 30 years of age; with age, the number of ephelides usually decreases. The main localization is on the face and hands, sometimes on the shoulders and torso.

Freckles are a manifestation of constitutive pigmentation, reflecting the distribution pattern of melanocytes in the skin, collected in "groups" rather than evenly distributed. The melanin protection of freckled skin can be compared to a hole in the sun, individuals with such skin need to avoid direct sunlight.

Melasma

Melasma is a symmetrically acquired melanin pigmentation on sun-exposed areas, most often on the face and neck, less often on the extensor surfaces of the shoulders and forearms, chest, and upper back. The spots' color varies from shades of brown (superficial pigment deposits) to bluish–gray (deep pigment deposits). Women aged 11–49 years (mean age 29.9 years) are most frequently affected. A distinction is made between centrofacial (forehead, cheeks, nasolabial fold, nose, and chin) (**Fig. II-5**), malar (cheeks and nose), and mandibular (mandibular region) melasma, and extrafacial melasma (**Fig. II-6**).

Causes include sun exposure and genetic predisposition. UV irradiation induces melanocortin production by melanocytes and keratino-

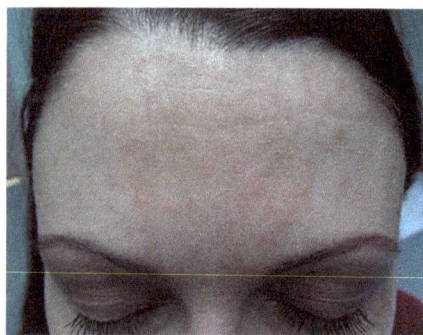

Figure II-5. Centrofacial melasma (Image by Albanova V.I.)

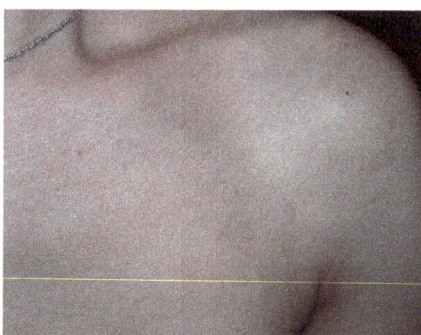

Figure II-6. Extrafacial melasma during administration of sex hormones (Image by Albanova V.I.)

cytes, increases blood circulation, causes skin inflammation, and forms a chronic photodamaged skin pattern. Hormones play an important role in this process. Melasma is most typical for pregnancy (in which case, it is often called chloasma). Contraceptives, hormone therapy, and endocrine disorders sometimes cause the disease. In some cases, melasma is induced by cosmetic products and topical photosensitizers. Sun exposure worsens the clinical picture.

It should be noted that recent studies have demonstrated the contribution of the vascular component in melasma development — the number, size, and density of blood vessels are higher in melasma-affected skin compared to the surrounding areas. Biopsy specimens from affected areas show increased numbers of mast cells that release many mediators, including histamine, VEGF, TNFα, and IL-8, which contribute to vascular proliferation.

Drug-induced pigmentation

Drug-induced pigmentation is associated with the use of oral or external photosensitizing drugs:

- Combined hormonal contraceptives
- Antibiotics — tetracyclines, sulfonamides, fluoroquinolones (1st and 2nd generations), griseofulvin (**Fig. II-7**)
- Cardiovascular drugs — antihypertensives, furosemide, amiodarone
- Non-steroidal anti-inflammatory drugs (NSAIDs) — pyroxicam

- Barbiturates
- Anti-tumor drugs — bleo-mycin, 5-fluorouracil
- Essential oils — berga-mot, citrus
- Coal tar
- Furocoumarins
- Psoralen

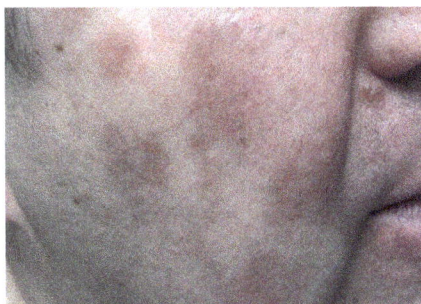

Figure II-7. Pigmentation after antibiotic administration (Image by Albanova V.I.)

Often patients must take some of these drugs for a long time. For example, minocycline (tetracycline antibiotic group) is a rheumatoid arthritis medication. Pigmentation occurs after 9–12 months of taking it; even if the drug use is discontinued, it persists for a long time.

Iron, multivitamin supplements containing ascorbic acid, advanced liver disease, and vitamin D deficiency reduce the risk of pigmentation (Hanada Y. et al., 2016).

Post-inflammatory pigmentation

Pigmentations accompany or appear in the final stages of many skin diseases; most often, they emerge alongside post-inflammatory processes such as:

- Acne (**Fig. II-8** and **II-9**)
- Psoriasis

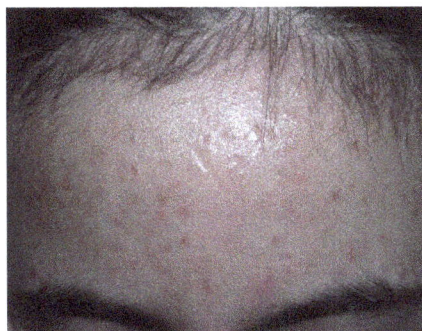

Figure II-8. Post-acne spots (Image by Albanova V.I.)

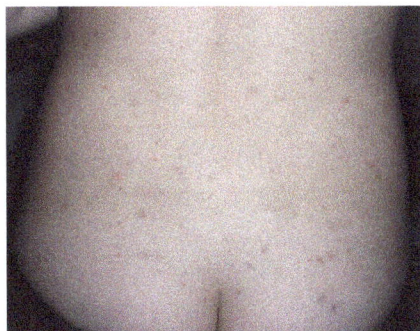

Figure II-9. Post-acne spots (Image byAlbanova V.I.)

- Atopic dermatitis (**Fig. II-10**)
- Pink lichen (lichen planus) (**Fig. II-11**)
- Contact allergic dermatitis (e.g., insect bites, jellyfish touch) (**Fig. II-12** and **II-13**)

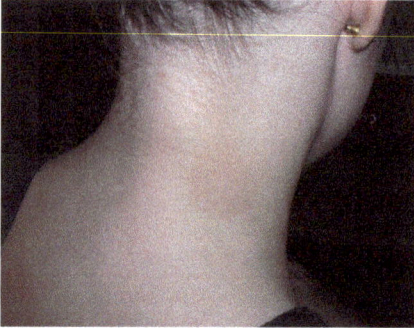

Figure II-10. Atopic dermatitis. Post-rash pigmentation on the neck (Image by Albanova V.I.)

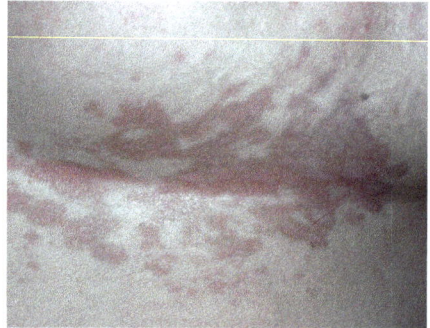

Figure II-11. Lichen planus. Persistent pigmentation (Image by Albanova V.I.)

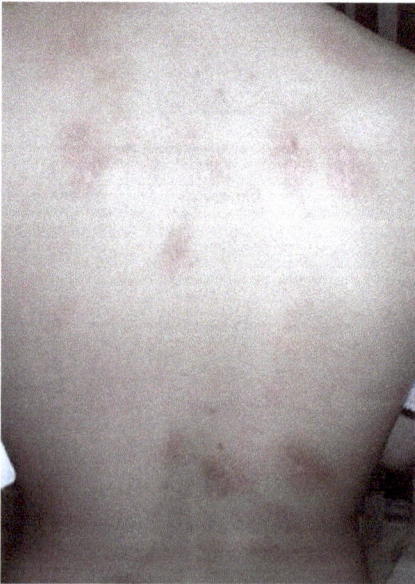

Figure II-12. Pigmentation on scratch sites in allergic dermatitis (Image by Albanova V.I.)

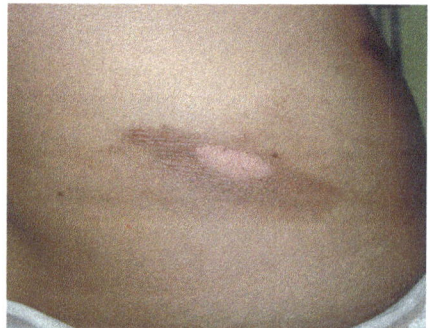

Figure II-13. Pigmentation after jellyfish stings (Image by Albanova V.I.)

- Autoimmune diseases
- Pyoderma (**Fig. II-14**)
- Bullous dermatoses
- Pigmented urticaria (mastocytosis) (**Fig. II-15**)
- Diaper rash
- Fungal diseases (pityriasis, dermatophytosis) (**Fig. II-16**)
- Viral diseases (shingles) (**Fig. II-17**)

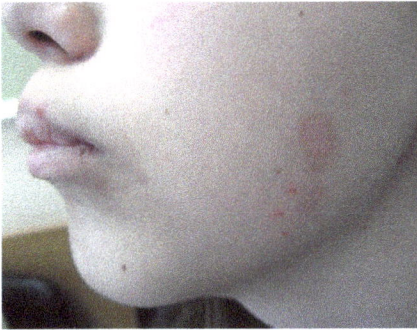

Figure II-14. Pigmentation after impetigo (Image by Albanova V.I.)

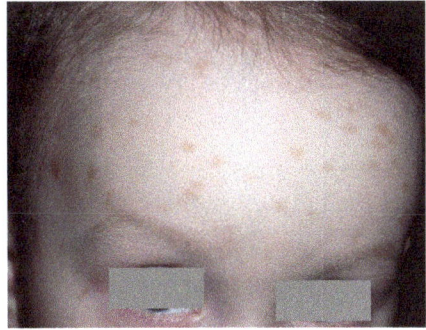

Figure II-15. Mastocytosis (Image by Albanova V.I.)

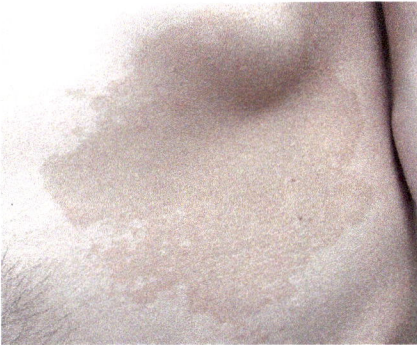

Figure II-16. Shingles (Image by Albanova V.I.)

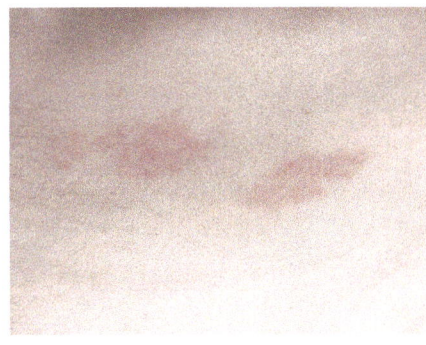

Figure II-17. Post-shingles pigmentation (Image by Albanova V.I.)

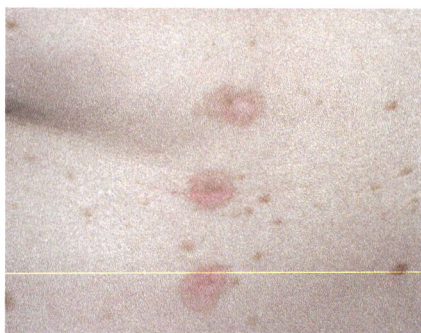

Figure II-18. Pigmentation after hirudotherapy (Image by Albanova V.I.)

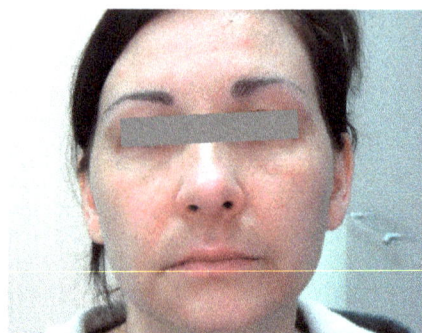

Figure II-19. Pigmentation after trichloroacetic acid peeling (Image by Albanova V.I.)

Most pigmentary disorders are related to external influences, such as:

- Tanning, radiation dermatitis
- Thermal and chemical burns
- Insect bites
- Jellyfish sting (**Fig. II-13**)
- Hirudotherapy (**Fig. II-18**)
- Contact with plants
- Skin-damaging aesthetic procedures (**Fig. II-19**)
- Topical medications
- Wounds, abrasions

Post-inflammatory pigmentations are always localized to the site of inflammation or rash. Sometimes, pigmentation occurs after complete resolution of the rash. On examination, the rash is not visible. A careful medical history collection helps to identify the nature of pigmentation. Skin darkening is more pronounced in chronic and recurrent inflammatory processes, as well as damage to the basal layer of the epidermis (Taylor S. et al., 2009; Achar A., Rathi S.K., 2011; Dantas L.P., Boza J.C., 2014).

Post-inflammatory pigmentation develops due to both increased melanin production and impaired melanin distribution. An increase in melanin can be caused by prostaglandins (E2 and D2), inflammatory cytokines (IL-1, IL-6, TNFα), some growth factors (EGF), and ROS. Pro-inflammatory cytokines, inflammatory mediators, and reactive oxygen species stimulate melanocyte growth, an increase in their outgrowth, and tyrosinase activity (Cestari T.F. et al., 2014). Like other pigmentations, post-inflammatory ones are more pronounced in people with darker skin.

Post-inflammatory pigmentation is typically localized in the epidermis (brown pigmentation). However, in some cases, when the epidermal basal cells and membrane are damaged, pigment enters the dermis and is taken up by macrophages. The pigmentation becomes deep and persistent, and the skin takes on a bluish–gray color, such as with squamous lichen (see **Fig. II-11**). Dermal pigmentation can persist for many years or even remain for life. Post-inflammatory pigmentation is exacerbated by exposure to UV light and recurrent inflammation.

Post-inflammatory pigmentations should be treated as early as possible, primarily taking care to resolve the inflammation. The main problem with post-inflammatory pigmentation, especially in people with dark skin, is skin irritation with bleaching ingredients, which can intensify pigmentation or even contribute to pigment "migration" into the dermis. Therefore, when used to correct post-inflammatory pigmentation, bleaching agents should be combined with anti-inflammatory and antioxidant medications, while ensuring full protection against UV radiation. However, while external agents effectively treat superficial pigmentations, deep pigmentations are poorly treated locally, and laser therapy is usually required in such cases (Davis E.C., Callender V.D., 2010).

Periorbital pigmentation

Periorbital hyperpigmentation can be physiological (familial, age-related) (**Fig. II-20**) or a symptom of various diseases (**Fig. II-21**).

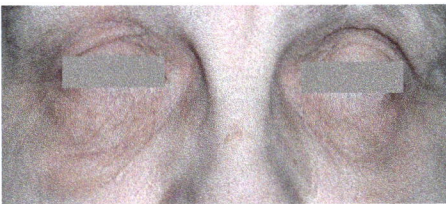

Figure II-20. Age-related periorbital hyperpigmentation (Image by Albanova V.I.)

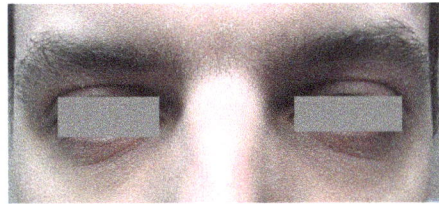

Figure II-21. Periorbital pigmentation in a patient with atopic dermatitis (Image by Albanova V.I.)

It is symmetrical, homogeneous, and located more often under the lower eyelids, but it can also involve the entire periorbital area. Its intensity depends on the organism's physiological state — it is more noticeable with fatigue, lack of sleep, and old age. As a symptom of skin diseases, it occurs in atopic dermatitis and allergies (especially to aeroallergens and medications). In these cases, it can be regarded as post-inflammatory due to rubbing and scratching the eyelids.

Phytophotodermatoses

Phytophotodermatoses result from contact with plants containing furocoumarins or psoralens. A phototoxic reaction develops because of subsequent sun exposure. The intensity of the reaction can vary depending on the plant, the phototype, and the duration of insolation. The most severe reactions are caused by milk thistle and birchweed. In erythema, small and large blisters appear on exposed skin areas that have come into contact with the plant, which may be accompanied by an impairment of the general condition. Pigmentation persists long after the rash has been resolved, and starts regressing in a few months. Unlike allergic reactions, phototoxic reactions are not accompanied by itching. Phototoxic reactions can be caused by members of the *Rutaceae* family (citrus fruits, mainly their peel — orange, lime, tangerine), *Apiacea* (carrot, celery, angelica, dill, parsley, anise, coriander), *Moraceae* (fig) (Cestari T.F. et al., 2014). Phototoxic reactions to bergamot oil (containing bergapten) included in some cosmetics compositions have also been reported.

Ashy dermatosis

Ashy dermatosis (*erythema dyschromicum perstans*) is characterized by symmetrical gray spots with indistinct boundaries on the trunk and proximal parts of the limbs. Sometimes mild erythema is detected at the edge of the spots. The causes of the disease are unknown.

1.1.3. Non-melanin-related skin color changes

Non-melanin-related skin color changes are ochronosis (alkaptonuria) and argyria. Exposure to mercury, bismuth, gold, arsenic, and antimalarial drugs can also change the skin color due to the accumulation of non-melanin dyes in the skin.

Ochronosis

Ochronosis (alkaptonuria) is an inherited defect of homogentisinic acid oxidase (homogentinase), which breaks down homogentisinic acid. The disease is more common in men than in women and mostly affects those aged 30–50 years. In ochronosis, the skin is grayish–brown, especially in the exposed areas, blue–green in the axillae, the nails are brittle and bluish, with brown streaks in the distal sections, dotted black pigmentation around the eyes, pigmented sclerae, complaints of numbness of the lumbosacral spine, black–brown urine, joint pain, deforming arthritis of the knee, less often of the hip joints.

There is also a variant of acquired ochronosis that occurs with prolonged use of hydroquinone.

Argyria

Argyria (argyrosis) — accumulation of silver in sweat and sebaceous glands, dermis, hair follicles, blood vessel walls, muscles, nervous tissue, mucous membranes, and internal organs. The color change is irreversible, and the development is gradual after several years of intake of silver salts. Prolonged external use of ointments and wound coatings containing silver compounds can also lead to persistent staining of the skin (local argyria).

Jaundice

Yellow skin can be a sign of disease and/or eating habits but can also occur as a result of certain medications. **Jaundice (true jaundice)** is a symptom complex characterized by yellowish staining of the skin and mucous membranes due to the accumulation of bilirubin in the tissues and blood. True jaundice may develop because of:
1. Excessive destruction of red blood cells and increased production of bilirubin — hemolytic (or suprahepatic) jaundice
2. Disorders in the bilirubin capture by liver cells and its binding to glucuronic acid — parenchymatous (or hepatic-cellular) jaundice
3. Obstruction of bilirubin excretion with bile into intestine — mechanical (or subhepatic) jaundice

False jaundice (pseudojaundice, carotene jaundice) — yellowish coloring of the skin (but not the mucous membranes) due to the accumulation of carotenes in it due to prolonged and abundant consumption of carrot, beet, orange, and pumpkin.

1.1.4. Hypomelanoses

Hypomelanoses (leucoderma, leucomelanosis) include albinism, vitiligo, post-inflammatory hypopigmentation, toxicoderma (after exposure to mercury, arsenic, phenol), idiopathic hypomelanosis, and pigmentless nevi. Such disorders associated with the reduction or disappearance of pigment are much more difficult to treat; congenital ones are not treatable.

Hypomelanoses can be associated either with a decrease in the number of melanocytes or with their normal content in the presence of a defect in the melanogenesis or melanosome transport system. For example, vitiligo is an idiopathic skin pigmentation disorder characterized by the appearance of well-defined depigmented/hypopigmented patches on the skin and mucosa. The etiology of vitiligo is not fully understood, but the leading role in damage to melanocytes and the disruption of melanogenesis is attributed to autoimmune mechanisms.

However, skincare specialists do not usually deal with hypomelanosis. They often see clients with facultative abnormal pigmentation, including post-inflammatory pigmentation, solar lentigo, and melasma.

1.2. Pigmentation analysis

Before you take on dyschromia treatment, you need to determine if the dyschromia is dangerous to your health. A **dermatoscope** helps the dermatologist to make this initial differential diagnosis. Dermatoscopy skills are also desirable for skincare specialists who work with pigmented blemishes. It is especially important for those professionals who perform laser removal of pigmentation. Naturally, if there is even the slightest suspicion, the patient should immediately be referred to a dermato-oncologist. Under no circumstances should any treatment be offered until the situation becomes clearer. If we are sure that the pigmented spot is not malignant, it can be treated using cosmetic methods.

The outcome of any bleaching method depends on the patient's ethnicity and the nature of the pigmentation (whether it is a manifestation of a pathological or physiological condition in this particular case). The therapy options for melanogenesis disorders also depend on which stages of the process are affected. When choosing a bleaching strategy, getting as detailed answers to the questions listed below is important.

1. Are melanocytes in their normal functional state, which is typical for this skin type, or are they overactive due to some factors?
2. Are the factors that caused the hyperpigmentation still present and can they be eliminated?
3. Is this pigmentation temporary, e.g., due to pregnancy, taking hormonal contraceptives, medications, etc.?
4. Is it possible to solve this problem without the use of dermatological drugs?
5. What area of skin will be treated?

To answer these questions, it is important to conduct a complete diagnosis based on the information obtained through an interview and subjective and objective examination of the patient.

1.2.1. Anamnesis

Important anamnestic data include duration and dynamics of pigmentation, a family tendency to pigmentation, presence of internal organ pathology, use of any medications (start and duration, change of dose, switching to another drug), harmful factors related to professional activity, insolation, exposure to different types of radiation, and any prior cosmetic procedures. During the examination, it is important to assess the phototype, localization, prevalence, outline, color, and symmetry of the location of hyperpigmentation foci.

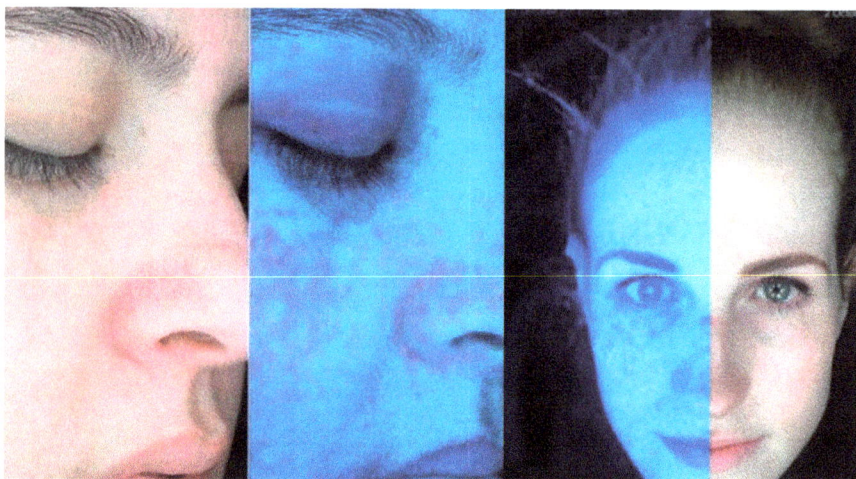

Figure II-22. Pigmentation analysis with the Wood lamp

1.2.2. Examination

In a dermatologist's practice, examination of patients with pigmentary defects includes dermatoscopy, examination with a Wood lamp, clinical blood tests, determination of zinc, copper, iron, and ferritin blood levels, and consultations with an endocrinologist and a therapist. If necessary, a skin biopsy is performed. Examination with a Wood lamp helps establish the depth of pigmentation: epidermal when there is a color enhancement, dermal when there is no enhancement (**Fig. II-22**). There is also a simple visual method: superficial defects are usually brown while deep defects are blue.

In all cases, it is useful to take photographs to compare symmetrical and intact areas and perform periodic evaluations during treatment.

1.2.3. Instrumental evaluation of pigmentation when planning aesthetic treatment

The devices for express pigmentation evaluation are now very popular. They are very useful for obtaining the information necessary for choosing the strategies for spot treatment quickly and non-invasively, namely:

1. Phototype (i.e., the basic activity of melanocytes)
2. Individual protection time (IPT): the speed of the skin's response to UV irradiation in the form of melanogenesis activation
3. Pigment amount in the skin
4. Depth of the pigment
5. Stain borders

The methods used for this purpose are described below.

Mexametry

The mexametry was developed by CK electronic GmbH (Germany) to quantify skin color, which largely depends on the content of two pigments — melanin and hemoglobin. The determination of hemoglobin is also important in diagnosing pigment disorders since some have a vascular component at their core.

Mexametry allows the contribution of each of these to be assessed separately, which is important for clinical practice. Moreover, subclinical erythema may not be visible on tanned or darkened skin, indicating a focus of inflammation. If it is present, the inflammation must be removed before the bleaching procedures or laser treatment. Otherwise, the skin may react through post-traumatic pigmentation. The mexameter probe allows you to accurately determine if there is inflammation beneath the pigmented spot (**Fig. II-23**).

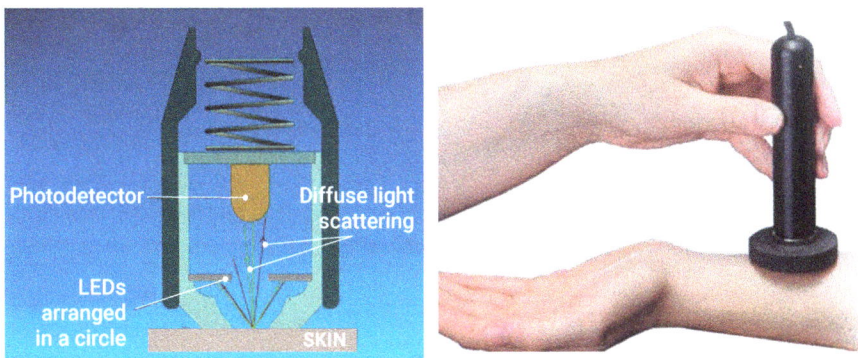

Figure II-23. Principle of Mexameter operation and measurements (CK electronic GmbH, Germany)

The method is based on the fact that melanin and hemoglobin absorb light differently. The sensor has 16 light-emitting diodes (LEDs) producing radiation at three wavelengths — 568 nm (green), 660 nm (red), and 870 nm (infrared). In the skin, the light is partially absorbed by melanin and hemoglobin, and the sensor on the photodetector captures its reflected part. Based on the analysis of the reflected spectrum, the amount of melanin and hemoglobin in each skin area is determined. The measurement result is given in two figures, which can be saved and used later to assess any changes in the skin condition over time. In addition, based on the measurements taken, objective recommendations are given for selecting sunscreens depending on the patient's phototype, overall health status, and climatic conditions.

In skincare practice, this method is used for:
1. Determining skin phototype and IPT to select the correct sunscreen product and tanning program in the tanning bed
2. Assessing the degree of erythema (inflammation)
3. Evaluating the effectiveness of whitening products and procedures

UV visualization

Melanin absorbs UV light well. Therefore, UV light is used to visualize pigmented areas of the skin. The absorbed radiation is not converted into visible fluorescence, and hidden photodamage and pigment spots become visible.

The prototype of modern photodiagnostic devices is the Wood lamp, a fluorescent device that emits UV light with a fundamental wavelength of 365 nm. Today, LEDs are used as a source of UV light, and special filters can polarize it (cross-polarization and parallel polarization modes), which expands the diagnostic capabilities. In particular, the cross-polarization mode is best for detecting pigmentary and vascular abnormalities (**Fig. II-24**).

As an example of photodiagnostic devices, the Observ 520 (Inno-Faith Beauty Science, the Netherlands) allows visualization of various skin conditions in six light modes, as well as Visioface 1000 (CK electronic GmbH, Germany). A person's head is fixed inside a hollow sphere with a blackout curtain, and then the illumination is turned on. Thanks

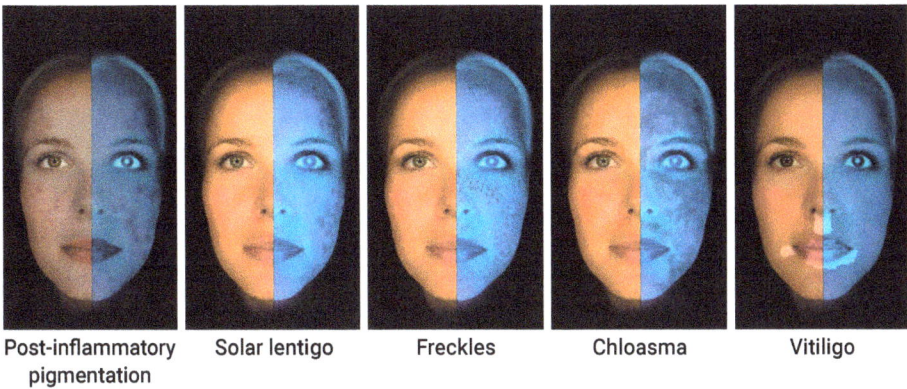

| Post-inflammatory pigmentation | Solar lentigo | Freckles | Chloasma | Vitiligo |

Figure II-24. Various pigment abnormalities in cross-polarized UV light Observ 520 (InnoFaith Beauty Science, the Netherlands)

to the additional mirror inside the sphere, not only the specialist, but also the patient can see the obtained picture. Moreover, the image can be photographed and saved to compare and evaluate the effectiveness of lightening agents in the future.

In the skincare practice, devices like Observ 520 and Visioface 1000 are used for:

- Determining the nature and extent of the damage
- Photodocumentation

3D visualization

The working principle of 3D imaging devices, such as Antera 3D (Miravex, Ireland), is also based on evaluating light absorption of different wavelengths generated by LEDs — but within the visible spectral range. In a few seconds, the device takes thousands of pictures of a selected area from different angles, views, and light intensities. This makes it possible to determine the amount and distribution of oxyhemoglobin, which has absorption peaks in the blue and yellow parts of the spectrum, as well as melanin, which is a good absorber of radiation in the green and red spectral range. Then special software analyzes the results and creates a 3D model of the skin surface, making it possible to assess the relief's condition and the distribution of pigment and vascular network (**Fig. II-25**).

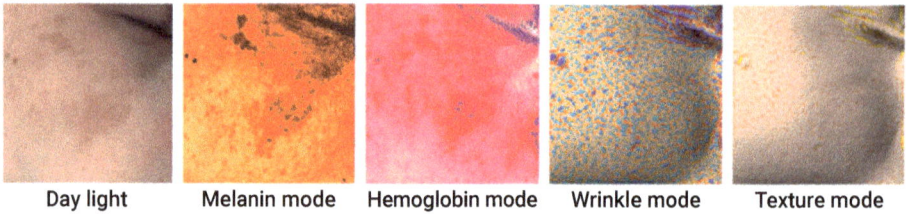

| Day light | Melanin mode | Hemoglobin mode | Wrinkle mode | Texture mode |

Figure II-25. Antera 3D operating modes (Miravex, Ireland)

Instrumental methods of skin assessment are an objective and reliable means at the skincare specialist's disposal with the following benefits:

1. Valuable information when choosing a method of pigmentation treatment, increasing its effectiveness and reducing the risks
2. Increasing customer loyalty
3. "Insurance policy" against unjustifiable claims from the client

1.3. What pigmentation types can an aesthetician work with?

Bleaching of physiologically dark skin (ethnic skin) has become a social phenomenon, much to doctors' concern. Because many people still consider white skin to be more attractive and even more "noble," women put their skin and their health at risk by trying to achieve a light tone that is unnatural for them. On the other hand, white Caucasians sometimes irrationally put their skin at risk by trying to achieve a darker tan. They also try to fight freckles, which are a manifestation of constitutive pigmentation, reflecting the distribution of melanocytes in the skin — only in this case, they gather in "groups" rather than being distributed evenly. This problem will probably only be solved when the last vestiges of racism and prejudice disappear from the planet and people finally realize that skin color, like hair color, is not a determining factor in beauty matters.

The persistent desire to make their skin lighter leads women to use strong bleaching products, regardless of the serious side effects. In response to this high demand, Asian and African manufacturers continue to produce depigmenting creams based on lead and mercury derivatives, despite numerous studies confirming their toxicity. Often, they do not inform buyers about the composition of their preparations and possible complications after use. This is highly problematic, given that 17 of the 38 randomly selected commercial whitening products tested in a study conducted in Saudi Arabia contained mercury.

In Europe and America, the production and sale of lightening products is much more strictly controlled. There is usually no lead or mercury in their composition. Still, a beautician taking on a client demanding ethnic skin brightening should remember that constitutional pigmentation is extremely difficult to bleach. There are significant risks involved in treating it.

It is much more expedient (from the biological point of view, which, alas, may not coincide with the patient's desires and preferences) for the skincare specialist to eliminate the consequences of pathological processes, to create conditions for the normal life of the skin cells, and to restore peace and harmony in the cellular state. If we approach whitening from these positions, the impact on the pigmentation in the skin should be as comprehensive and gentle as possible. Unfortunately, constitutive pigmentation is impossible to whiten. The skin that one tries to deprive of its natural protection resists with all its might, so heavy artillery must be used, and it does not always work "cleanly and silently."

It is also necessary to consider the size of the surface area treated with bleaching medications, which can be large when lightening dark ethnic skin and significantly increases the risk of complications. It is one thing to damage melanocytes in a small area and quite another to expose the entire face or a large area of the body to toxic effects. Since it is very difficult to change the genetically determined level of melanin synthesis for any appreciable period, it should be understood that the patient will have to regularly undergo the whitening procedures. This runs the risk of both premature skin aging and the development of permanent pigmentation disorders, such as hypopigmentation, which are virtually uncorrectable.

Sometimes we have to deal with pathological pigmentation of dark skin or the task of whitening dark skin to reduce contrast in vitiligo. In these cases, it should be remembered that increased pigmentation is the skin's natural response to damage. Therefore, using agents that irritate or damage the skin can also lead to a paradoxical increase in pigmentation. For example, the use of lasers and deep (or even medi-um-depth) peels to eliminate abnormal pigmentation of dark skin or to reduce contrast in vitiligo can lead to the development of hyperpig-mentation, even when all the necessary measures to protect against UV radiation have been followed.

Part III

Aesthetic methods for preventing and treating pigment spots

Melanogenesis is a complex and finely balanced process that involves all skin cells and many of the signaling pathways we discussed in the preceding parts of this book. This entire production–logistics chain comes into motion after stress (e.g., UV light, trauma, hormonal disorders) and represents a variant of the skin's adaptive reaction aimed at strengthening its own protective structures (in this case, photoprotection in the form of increasing the amount of melanin on the "weakened" area is enhanced).

Theoretically, it is possible to interfere with this process both at the production and transport stages. Practically, it is extremely difficult to do so. There is too much intertwining with other defense systems, including antioxidant and immune mechanisms. Alas, we must admit: in the fight against hyperpigmentation, it is difficult to be an absolute winner, although modern skincare methods sometimes allow it (Serre C. et al., 2018). In addition, as we have already mentioned, it is not only melanin that is involved in the formation of skin color, giving the skin different shades of brown tone. Hemoglobin combined with oxygen (oxyhemoglobin) gives the skin a bright red hue and, in its reduced form (deoxyhemoglobin), it gives a blue hue. Carotenoids color skin yellow (β-carotene and lutein) and orange (lycopene). Moisture saturation of the skin, the state of dermal collagen, gender, age, wrinkles, and regional skin characteristics also play a role. All these components contribute to the evenness of skin tone.

Before you start treating a pigmented defect, you need to establish a diagnosis and try to understand the causes and the likelihood of eliminating them. Sometimes, in addition to a dermatologist, a dermato-oncologist and endocrinologist are involved. In some cases, pigmentation is temporary and can resolve on its own after eliminating the factors that caused it, such as pregnancy, taking combined oral contraceptives (OCs), or certain medications. **Before starting treatment, it is important to make sure that the patient's problem has a solution at all.** For example, in the case of dermally pigmented squamous lesions, using any means or methods is unlikely to produce the desired result.

Even if there are realistic ways of achieving beneficial results, subjective factors should be evaluated, making sure that the patient is ready for long-term treatment (which always takes several months). Even if the patient can follow the doctor's instructions exactly and achieve results, it is important to observe the rules of prevention of relapse since sun protection will be required for a very long time, and its absence will quickly nullify all the successes achieved. It is also necessary to discuss the financial costs with the patient, providing a treatment plan and the approximate prices of all its components.

In many cases, the treatment of pigmentation is beyond the scope of skincare specialists, and medical consultation is necessary. As we have already mentioned, if there is the slightest suspicion of a malignant skin neoplasm, the patient should be referred to a dermato-on-cologist. Consultation with a physician is also necessary for skin pigmentation caused by internal diseases.

The anti-pigmentation program available to the skincare specialist involves depigmenting, brightening, anti-inflammatory, antioxidant, and sunscreen products and techniques.

Methods that directly affect the process of melanogenesis in its various stages are called depigmenting (or whitening). They include:
- Topical depigmentants (Shah S., Chew S.K., 2018; Pillaiyar T. et al., 2018)
- Selective photothermolysis (Mei X.L., Wang L., 2018)

In contrast to depigmenting methods, lightening methods smooth the skin surface, changing its optical properties by:
- Exfoliation (chemical peeling, microdermabrasion, laser resurfacing)
- Moistening of the *stratum corneum*
- Wrinkle filling with cosmetic preparations containing so-called optical pigments, which change the light scattering properties of the skin surface (giving the effect of radiance and brightening)

All the above methods are used to lighten hyperpigmentation that is already present. However, if success is achieved, it does not last long if the causative agents are not removed. Therefore, it is extremely important to address three more points:

1. **Reduce UV exposure** — this is the main factor that stimulates pigmentation, so the use of sunscreens with a high degree of protection (SPF > 30) is mandatory throughout the treatment period
2. **Remove inflammation** (it produces ROS as the main melanogenesis triggers) — use antioxidant, anti-inflammatory, and soothing agents
3. **Strengthen the barrier structures of the *stratum corneum*** by using moisturizers and emollients

Once again, photoprotection measures are a prerequisite for all whitening procedures. As the treated skin areas become more vulnerable to UV damage, clients should be advised to avoid direct sunlight and use special sunscreens.

In addition, since the effects of UV light, air pollutants, and any inflammatory processes are associated with ROS formation, to reduce the risk of stimulating melanogenesis, antioxidants should be introduced into the course of pigmentation treatment and skincare in general. Like sunscreens, they should be started before using aggressive depigmenting and lightening agents and methods.

Thus, the general approach to the pigmentation treatment is to perform the following set of actions:

1. Reduce the background activity of melanocytes by removing the factors that provoke pigmentation with sunscreens, anti-pollution, antioxidants, and anti-inflammatory formulations to block the melanin formation and distribution in the skin or destroy the pigment with depigmenting agents and methods
2. Accelerate the elimination of existing melanin with lightening agents and methods that accelerate exfoliation
3. Provide protection and restoration of the skin's barrier functions

Chapter 1
Cosmetic products

1.1. Depigmenting and lightening agents

1.1.1. Targets in the skin

As mentioned previously, true depigmenting (bleaching) agents include substances that inhibit melanogenesis. Some act as competitive tyrosinase inhibitors, some block the synthesis of this enzyme, and others prevent the transfer of melanosomes from melanocytes to neighboring keratinocytes. However, most "work" on several fronts at the same time.

Exfoliating products can help lighten and even out the overall skin tone. Their purpose is to speed up the desquamation of melanin-overloaded corneocytes. Thus, if they simultaneously reduce melanin synthesis, new corneocytes will have less pigment and the skin will become lighter.

Retinol-based cosmetics and superficial chemical peels (hydroxy acids, keratolytic and enzymatic peels) are lightening products. It is currently not recommended to use medium-depth and deep peels to treat pigmentation lesions because aggressive skin damage can provoke pigmentation. When using peels to lighten skin with post-inflammatory pigmentation or ethnic skin, anti-inflammatory drugs must be used, and significant skin irritation must be avoided. Also, when considering peels in general, salicylic acid, which refer to beta-hydroxy acids, is not recommended on low-sebum skin.

According to the mechanism of action, all currently known depigmenting agents can be divided into two main groups:

1. **Toxic (non-specific):** Usually damage and kill melanocytes/ keratinocytes and destroy the mature melanin. Almost all

long-known bleaching agents traditionally used in dermatology belong to this group. For example, mercury and phenol compounds, hydroquinone, and azelaic acid can also have similar properties.

2. **Selective (specific):** Selectively inhibit either the activity of enzymes involved in melanogenesis or cell receptors perceiving the signal to enhance melanin synthesis. This group includes bleaching agents of the latest generation.

Currently, trends are increasingly moving away from the depigmentation methods that, while effective, are dangerous to the health of the skin and the body, giving preference to modern means and a comprehensive approach. The targets for skin lightening and approaches to pigmentation control are outlined in **Fig. III-1-1** and **III-1-2**.

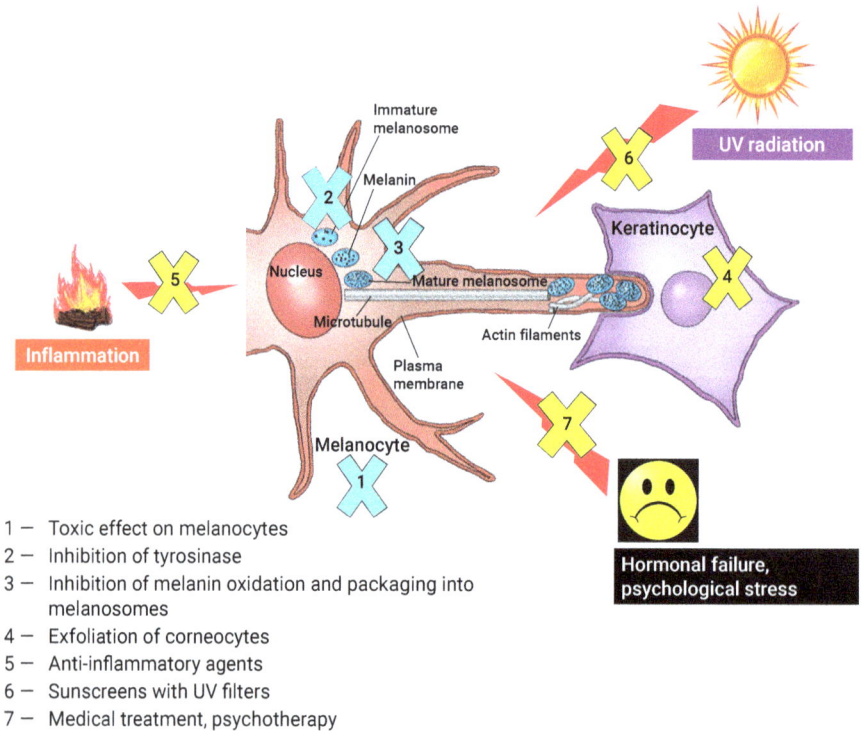

1 — Toxic effect on melanocytes
2 — Inhibition of tyrosinase
3 — Inhibition of melanin oxidation and packaging into melanosomes
4 — Exfoliation of corneocytes
5 — Anti-inflammatory agents
6 — Sunscreens with UV filters
7 — Medical treatment, psychotherapy

Figure III-1-1. Targets and aesthetic tools for skin lightening: 1–3 (blue) — direct melanogenesis inhibition; 4–7 (yellow) — indirect pigmentation reduction

PIGMENTATION CONTROL

DIRECT MELANOGENESIS INHIBITION	INDIRECT PIGMENTATION REDUCTION
■ Depigmenting agents: 1. Tyrosinase inhibitions 2. Pigment destruction ■ Melanin-loaded corneocyte exfoliation	■ Sunscreens with UV filters ■ Anti-inflammatory measures ■ Hormonal imbalance treatment ■ Psychotherapy

Figure III-1-2. An integrated approach to effective pigmentation control

Table III-1-1 lists the major groups of substances that are found in products used to correct pigmentation, both pharmaceutical and cosmetic. Plant extracts are not included in the table because they are mixtures of different substances, but they are discussed later when each substance is analyzed separately. **The more targets we involve in our treatment program, the better the chance of achieving the desired result!**

1.1.2. Obsolete and dangerous substances

The substances discussed in this section were previously routinely used for skin whitening. Although they are now banned due to toxicity, they can still be found on the market and thus deserve due attention in this book.

Mercury

In modern medicine, mercury is not considered a medicinal substance because it is a toxic metal with many proven negative effects. However, it has been used for centuries to whiten skin, and unfortunately, it is still used in some countries.

The whitening mechanism of mercury ions is rarely a subject of scientific research, but there is sufficient, albeit indirect, evidence that mercury causes severe oxidative stress at the melanocyte level. So, the toxic effect of mercury on melanocytes can be rightly called

Table III-1-1. The most common ingredients in formulations used for treating pigmentation

MAIN (BUT NOT THE ONLY) TARGET	SUBSTANCES
Inhibition of melanogenesis at different stages (true depigmenting substances)	
Cytotoxic effect	• Hydroquinone • Azelaic acid
Inhibits the synthesis of the amino acid tyrosine from precursors	• N-acetylglycosamine
Tyrosinase inhibition	• Hydroquinone • Arbutin • Kojic acid • Cinnamic acid
Inhibition of melanosome transfer to keratinocytes	• Soybean enzymes • Niacinamide
Reducing agents (prevent oxidative processes, in the course of which ready melanin is produced)	• Ascorbic acid
Melanosome destruction	• Hydrogen peroxide • Lignin peroxidase
Prevention of melanogenesis or reduction of its intensity (substances that create conditions conducive to the melanocyte activity reduction)	
Binding of metal ions of variable valence (copper, iron), which are initiators of free-radical chain reactions	• EDTA • Azelaic acid • Phytic acid
Reducing inflammation	• Antioxidants (e.g., plant polyphenols)
Elimination of the consequences of increased melanogenesis (substances that reduce the amount of pigment by accelerating corneocyte exfoliation)	
Exfoliating	• Alpha hydroxy acids (AHAs) • Salicylic acid • Retinol

"disarming" because mercury ions non-selectivly inhibit all antioxi-dant systems designed to protect melanocytes from free-radical "ex-plosion." Another hypothesis for their mode of action implicates ty-rosinase inhibition.

The problem is that mercury from bleaching products can be ab-sorbed through the skin and accumulate in various organs, causing marked nephro- and neurotoxic effects. A separate problem is that cosmetic products with mercury have been used primarily not to cor-rect pitting hyperpigmentation but to lighten skin tone in general by residents of southern countries. Mercury use is now officially banned due to its toxic effects, but unfortunately, mercury-containing prod-ucts are still being used by dark-skinned people, mostly in developing countries. As a result, reports of mercury intoxication continue to ap-pear in academic publications (Kuehn B., 2020).

Phenol compounds

The depigmenting effect of phenolic compounds was first noted in workers who wore rubber gloves impregnated with benzoic hydroqui-none ester to protect their hands from oxidation. Numerous phenol derivatives, such as cresol, hydroquinone, and benzoic hydroquinone ester, have a similar effect.

The mechanism of phenols' action is associated with free radicals of these compounds — semiquinones, formed on the enzyme tyrosi-nase. Due to subsequent reactions, they give rise to a whole family of reactive oxygen species with "killing potential" against melanocytes and keratinocytes. It is very important that the stability of semiquinone radicals (i.e., their ability to "rotate" in the redox cycle for a long time and efficiently) entirely determines the positive result of whitening. It is fundamentally important that semiquinone radicals of phenols can also be formed spontaneously, without the participation of the tyrosinase enzyme, especially in an acidic environment. However, in this case, their concentration is much lower than in the presence of the enzyme. Cur-rently, the use of phenol in cosmetics is banned in most countries.

Hydroquinone

Hydroquinone, also related to phenolic compounds, is one of the most widely recognized inhibitors of melanogenesis owing to its ability to markedly reduce tyrosinase activity due to its structural similarity with melanin precursors, "framing" itself under the action of the enzyme (Parvez S. et al., 2006; Deri B. et al., 2016). In addition, hydroquinone exhibits selective toxicity to melanocytes, damages melanosomes, and reversibly inhibits DNA and RNA synthesis (Penney K.B. et al., 1984). Semiquinone radicals released by the interaction of hydroquinone with tyrosinase have a damaging effect. The higher the concentration of hydroquinone in bleaching agents, the stronger its effect on melanocytes, but the higher the probability of free radical damage to skin cells. Moreover, as the dose increases, other skin cells can also be damaged.

Hydroquinone is combined with tretinoin and/or glycolic acid (due to its exfoliating action, they improve the penetration of hydroquinone) and corticosteroids (reduction of inflammation) to increase effectiveness and reduce the concentration and use duration — a combination known as the Kligman formula.

With prolonged hydroquinone use, allergic and contact dermatitis, cataracts, post-inflammatory hyperpigmentation, hypopigmentation of adjacent normal skin, loss of skin elasticity, nail pigmentation, and impaired wound healing may occur.

Since hydroquinone penetrates well through the skin and can be absorbed into the blood, it should not be used during pregnancy and lactation. There is also evidence — although obtained in animals and based on oral and injected intake — of carcinogenicity, nephrotoxicity, and effects on the reproductive system in rats. Topical use of the compound in rodents has been associated with increased skin tumor incidence. However, there are no clear data on similar effects in humans (McGregor D., 2007).

People with dark skin who use hydroquinone frequently and regularly over a long period may develop a rare complication, ochronosis. Although this condition rarely occurs in Europe and the United States, as hydroquinone is used extensively in Asian and African countries, ochronosis has become a serious problem in these populations. Hydroquinone inhibits the activity of homogentisic acid oxidase, a metabolite of tyrosine. Normally, it is rapidly destroyed, but with prolonged blockade of the enzyme that oxidizes it, homogentisic acid can accumulate in the dermal layer and polymerize to form a yellowish pigment. The first sign of ochronosis is coarsening and darkening of the skin in the areas treated with hydroquinone. Histological examination reveals yellow granules in the intercellular substance of the dermis (**ochronosis** — from the word "ochre"). In advanced ochronosis cases, skin atrophy and degeneration of elastin fibers occur because the pigment is deposited in and around them. There is also evidence of ochronosis of the eyes with long-term use of hydroquinone cream, including in the periorbital area (Hollick E.J. et al., 2019). Since 2001, the use of cosmetics with hydroquinone has been completely restricted in the European Union. Hydroquinone use in cosmetics has also been banned in Japan, Australia, and some African countries. The U.S. Food and Drug Administration (FDA) proposed banning over-the-counter cosmetic products with hydroquinone in 2006, but this ban is still not in force, although restrictions have been introduced. For example, in over-the-counter products, hydroquinone concentration cannot exceed 2%, while in prescription products, the limit is 4%.

Although hydroquinone is still actively used by consumers, most experts are gradually moving away from its use.

1.1.3. Active substances in modern topical pigmentation correctors

Let's take a closer look at the most common active ingredients in today's topical pigmentation-treating products.

Azelaic acid

Azelaic acid (1,7-heptandicarboxylic acid) is well-known to dermatologists as a treatment for acne. Studies have shown it is a weak direct inhibitor of tyrosinase (pronounced inhibition only in cytotoxic concentrations). However, azelaic acid is characterized by another indirect way of action on tyrosinase. It stimulates the activity of the enzyme thioredoxin reductase, which restores oxidized thioredoxin, an endogenous tyrosinase inhibitor. In addition, just like hydroquinone, azelaic acid inhibits DNA and RNA synthesis in melanocytes. It is also a chelator of metal ions of different valences (such as iron) that can trigger peroxidation chain reactions, activate melanogenesis, and exhibit anti-inflammatory and keratolytic activity.

Azelaic acid in the form of 15% gel or 20% cream is used to treat melasma and post-inflammatory pigmentation in acne. A comparison of the effectiveness of azelaic acid with hydroquinone in the treatment of melasma showed no significant difference (Balina L.M., Graupe K., 1991). In this study, after using 20% azelaic acid for 24 weeks, 64.8% of the participants reported good to excellent results. Using 4% hydroquinone for the same period provided similar effects in 72% of patients. In some cases, the combination of glycolic and azelaic acids may cause burning, scaling, and reddening of the skin, but the severity of these symptoms is negligible.

Arbutin

Arbutin (β-D-glucopyranoside hydroquinone) is a product of hydroquinone glycosylation. It is found in significant amounts in bearberry leaves, long used as a bleaching agent, and in some other plants, although not all have depigmenting action. Blueberries and lingonberries also contain arbutin.

Arbutin attracted the attention of cosmetics manufacturers after experiments showed its ability to inhibit melanin synthesis without having a toxic effect on melanocytes and other skin cells, only slightly reducing melanocyte activity. In human melanoma cell culture, arbutin at a concentration of 0.05 mM significantly reduced tyrosinase activity, and the melanin content in the cells decreased by 39%. However, therapy with arbutin must be prolonged — lasting weeks or even months — to achieve the desired effect. Arbutin has some antioxidant properties and improves skin recovery after photodamage (Zhou H. et al., 2019). The effectiveness of arbutin as a brightening agent increases with increasing concentration, although too high a concentration can exacerbate pigmentation. Synthetic forms of arbutin, α-arbutin and deoxyarbutin, characterized by a more pronounced ability to inhibit tyrosinase, are also used in cosmetic dermatology (Boissy R.E. et al., 2005). However, it is worth noting that both arbutin and deoxyarbutin can be converted into hydroquinone — especially under the influence of UVB radiation. Moreover, the use of 3% creams with deoxyarbutin has been associated with an "alarming" increase in hydroquinone levels in the skin, so the European Scientific Committee on Consumer Safety considers it unsafe to use this ingredient in cosmetics (SCCS,

Degen G.H., 2016). The transformation of arbutin into hydroquinone is slow, so its oxidative cytotoxic effects are low, although it is still not recommended to introduce arbutin into cosmetic formulations without antioxidants.

Kojic acid

Kojic acid (5-hydroxy-2-hydroxymethyl-4-pyrone) is also a tyrosinase inhibitor — it binds copper in the enzyme. In addition, it has an exfoliating effect, can bind divalent iron ions, and intercept free radicals. Among modern bleaching agents, kojic acid rivals hydroquinone and arbutin in popularity but is inferior to them in effectiveness. Typically, kojic acid is used in 1–4% concentration, as lower amounts have almost no effect. Often, kojic acid is combined with other depigmenting and brightening agents.

The main disadvantage of kojic acid is its potential allergenicity. Therefore, before using kojic acid preparations, a test should be carried out on the elbow bend. At the first sign of dermatitis, its use should be discontinued.

Ascorbic acid

Ascorbic acid (γ-lactone 2,3-dehydro-L-gulonic acid, vitamin C) is a strong reducing agent, inhibiting melanogenesis by reducing DOPA-chrome to DOPA-quinone. It also inhibits melanogenesis by interacting with copper ions, which are necessary for melanin synthesis, and blocks DHICA oxidation. Nevertheless, it was impossible to use ascorbic acid as a bleaching agent for a long time since it is extremely unstable and easily oxidized in its pure form, and most of its stable analogs do not penetrate the skin well.

Stable forms of ascorbic acid, such as ascorbyl-2-magnesium phosphate and ascorbyl-6-palmitate are now used in whitening products. Whitening cosmetics based on 0.3–3.0% ascorbyl-2-magnesium phosphate are recommended for evening the skin tone of young patients and improving the condition of aging skin with pigment spots.

An additional advantage of ascorbic acid preparations is their antioxidant activity and the ability to stimulate collagen synthesis in the skin. Like all acids, ascorbic acid-based bleaching agents can cause skin irritation.

Niacinamide

Niacinamide (3-pyridine-carboxamide, nicotinamide) is a physiologically active form of vitamin B_3 (niacin, nicotinic acid, vitamin PP). Niacinamide inhibits the transport of melanosomes into keratinocytes without affecting tyrosinase activity. There is speculation that niacinamide can also affect the cell crosstalk between keratinocytes and melanocytes so that keratinocytes begin to send a signal to melanocytes to reduce melanin synthesis. In addition, it has pronounced antioxidant and anti-inflammatory effect, improves skin barrier function by activating the synthesis of keratin, filaggrin, and involucrin, and stimulates fibroblast function (Chhabra G. et al., 2019).

Niacinamide is used in 2–5% concentrations, sometimes in combination with N-acetylglycosamine. The main advantages of niacinamide are its stability and safety. However, its efficacy is lower than that of hydroquinone and kojic acid.

N-acetylglycosamine

N-acetylglycosamine reduces melanin content in melanocytes by inhibiting the conversion of tyrosine precursors to tyrosine. Clinical studies show that 2% N-acetylglycosamine applied for eight weeks reduces facial pigmentation. It is commonly used in combination with niacinamide due to their synergistic effect.

Tranexamic acid

Tranexamic acid is a relatively new product in the cosmetics industry but has long been known in surgery. It is a synthetic derivative of the amino acid lysine and is used as a styptic and an anti-allergic and anti-inflammatory agent. Observing patients taking tranexamic acid, experts noticed that their skin became lighter.

Subsequent studies have shown that tranexamic acid affects several targets in the fight against hyperpigmentation, an already known anti-inflammatory effect, and causes a decrease in the sensitivity of melanocytes to pro-inflammatory agents in general. It also directly inhibits tyrosinase and melanin transfer (Kim M.S. et al., 2015). In addition, tranexamic acid reduces the level of pro-inflammatory arachidonic acid in keratinocytes in the UV-exposed skin. It inhibits prostaglandin production, thus inhibiting UV-induced melanogenesis and neovascularization (mediated inhibition of angiogenic fibroblast growth factor also plays a role here). It can also stimulate melanocyte autophagy (Cho Y.H. et al., 2017). At the same time, tranexamic acid is non-toxic and does not irritate even hypersensitive skin, unlike many depigmenting agents (George A., 2016).

A recent study compared the efficacy of treating melasma (mostly mixed) with a 5% tranexamic acid solution and a 3% hydroquinone cream. The agents were applied once a day for 12 weeks, and sunscreen was mandatory. Although the degree of skin lightening in both groups was similar, satisfaction was much higher in the tranexamic acid group due to significantly fewer side effects (Janney M.S. et al., 2019).

Lignin peroxidase (lignase)

Lignin peroxidase (lignase) is an enzyme found in wood-destroying fungi (*Phanerochaete chrysosporium*) that breaks down lignin, a poly-phenolic substance deposited in the shells of plant cells, causing them to become woody and increasing their strength. After a tree dies, lignin peroxidase splits lignin, which is structurally similar to melanin, resulting in discoloration and wood tissue loosening. Lignin peroxidase is used in the papermaking industry to lighten wood pulp for paper production. Due to its structural proximity, lignin peroxidase can oxidize and degrade melanin. Importantly, lignin peroxidase specifically destroys already prepared melanin without disrupting the complex mechanism of its biosynthesis. The enzyme is inactivated and destroyed in the skin naturally. Physiological "control" of the enzyme by the skin prevents systemic action and increases skin tolerance.

Cinnamic acid

Cinnamic acid (β-phenylacrylic acid, benzylidene acetic acid) is a phenyl propanol derivative, a polyphenol group precursor. It inhibits tyrosinase, has powerful antioxidant properties, and can absorb UVB radiation. It is used in sunscreens but is a photosensitizer and can cause photoallergic reactions.

Ferulic acid

Ferulic acid is one of the most powerful natural antioxidants. Its strength has been compared to that of superoxide dismutase. It gets its name from the perennial umbrella herb ferulic acid but is found in many fruits and plants, such as rice, wheat, oat bran, apple, coffee (beans) etc. Ferulic acid plays a key role in plants' self-preservation mechanism by increasing the cell wall's strength and protecting it from microbial damage and sun exposure — it can directly absorb quanta of UVB radiation (Peres D.D. et al., 2018). Therefore, unlike many other compounds, its activity not only does not decline but rather increases under the sun's influence.

In addition to its pronounced antioxidant, anti-inflammatory, immunomodulatory, and sun protection properties, ferulic acid exhibits some depigmentation activity. It has been shown to be able to inhibit melanin synthesis, tyrosinase expression, and expression of MITF — the α-MSH signaling molecule. Moreover, ferulic acid stimulates the synthesis of hyaluronic acid, collagen, and the tissue inhibitor of metalloproteinase synthesis, and inhibits the expression of MMP-1 and MMP-9 (Park H.J. et al., 2018).

Glycolic acid

Glycolic acid is not a depigmenting but a lightening agent. Like other AHAs (lactic acid, citric acid), it accelerates epidermis regeneration and is often used in hyperpigmentation programs to exfoliate the upper skin layers containing pigment.

Resveratrol

Resveratrol, another powerful antioxidant, was first isolated from dark grapes and grape seeds. In addition to its antioxidant effects, resveratrol can activate the *SIRT1* gene that encodes the sirtuin protein, an enzyme that modifies the histones on which DNA is wound. Through histones, sirtuins can influence the expression of genes, particularly the *p53* gene, the activation of which leads to apoptosis. In this way, sirtuins prolong cell life. Resveratrol improves respiratory processes in cells and has vasodilatory, anti-allergic, anti-inflammatory, radioprotective, and immunomodulatory effects. In addition, resveratrol affects several parts of melanogenesis simultaneously: as an alternative substrate for tyrosinase, it decreases its melanogenic activity and supresses tyrosinase-coding gene transcription. Besides, it reduces UV damage to keratinocytes and inhibits their signaling activity, which, in turn, helps regulate melanocyte function and generally reduces melanin synthesis (Na J.I. et al., 2019).

Fatty acids

Interestingly, unsaturated fatty acids can also regulate melanogenesis. For example, oleic, linoleic, and α-linolenic acids suppress tyrosinase activity and, therefore, melanogenesis, while palmitic and stearic acids increase it. Linoleic acid also affects skin pigmentation by stimulating epidermal renewal and increasing the desquamation of cells containing melanin (Ebanks J.P. et al., 2009).

1.1.4. Plant extracts with a complex lightening effect

Most of the substances discussed thus far are synthesized by plants. Often, they are included in the formulation of a topical remedy as part of plant extracts. Let us name the most popular plant sources.

Licorice

Licorice (*Glycyrrhiza glabra*) root extract is included in many whitening products. The main components of a licorice root extract that act on pigmentation are glabridine and liquiritin. Glabridine inhibits tyrosinase, and liquiritin acts by increasing the dispersion of melanin. They also have pronounced anti-inflammatory, antimicrobial, and antioxidant properties. Numerous studies have demonstrated their effectiveness against UVB-induced damage and pigmentation (including aggravation of epidermal melasma), comparable with hydroquinone, and in some cases superior to it (Zubair S., Mujtaba G., 2009; Makino E.T. et al., 2013).

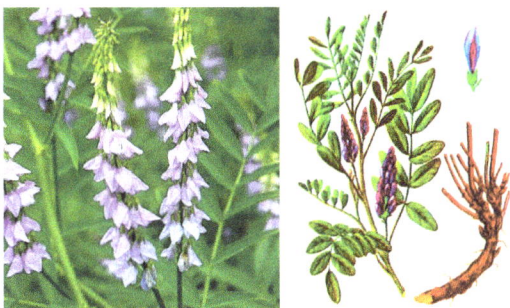

Glycyrrhiza glabra

Soybean

Some soybean proteins, such as trypsin and serine protease inhibitors, have an affinity for receptors on the keratinocyte membrane involved in melanosome transfer. As a result, the transfer of the melanosomes from melanocytes to keratinocytes is inhibited, and the skin pigment content is reduced. Soybean extract also has antioxidant and photoprotective activity. The protein fraction of soybean extract is combined with other lightening agents, retinoids, and sunscreens.

Mulberry

White mulberry (*Morus alba*) bark and root extracts exhibit depigmenting properties by inhibiting tyrosinase and melanosome tracer. They are also "catchers" of superoxide anion radicals and have an anti-inflammatory effect.

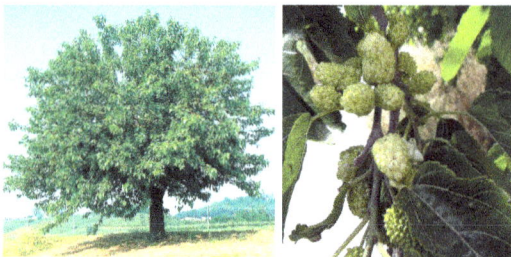

Morus alba

Aloe

Aloesin and aloin are the active ingredients of *Aloe vera* leaves, characterized by their lightening effect. Aloesin inhibits tyrosinase, tyrosine hydroxylase, and DOPA oxidase with no toxic effects, while aloin causes aggregation of melanin granules, which leads to skin lightening. Aloe extract is usually included in whitening compositions and other lightening and depigmenting ingredients (good effects are particularly noted when combined with arbutin).

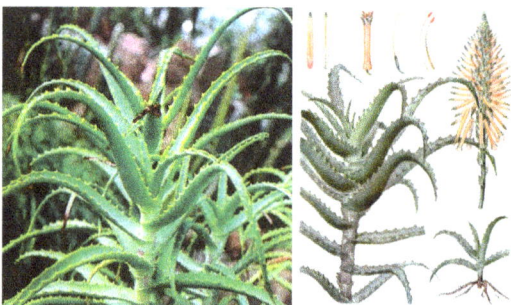

Aloe vera

Green tea

Green tea extract contains polyphenolic compounds with pronounced anti-inflammatory and antioxidant properties. In addition, epigallo-catechin-3-gallate (ECGC), which can inhibit tyrosinase, has a depigmenting effect. Green tea extract can also suppress UV-induced erythema, reduce sunburn, and protect DNA from UV radiation.

Shiitake mushrooms

Shiitake mushrooms (*Lentinus edodes*) are highly prized in Asia for their medicinal properties. Scientific studies have shown that shiitake extract contains kojic acid, which is associated with its whitening effect. The most notable component of shiitake mushrooms is the polysaccharide lentinan (β-1,3-glucan), which has pronounced immune-stimulating and anti-inflammatory properties. In addition, shiitake extract has been shown to stimulate collagen synthesis.

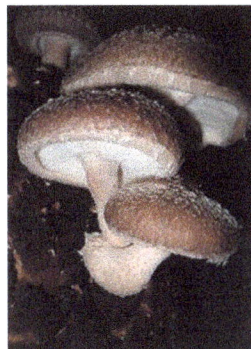

Lentinus edodes

1.1.5. Retinoids

Retinoids — structural or functional analogues of vitamin A — were originally used "to help" hydroquinone in Kligman's formula. Gradually their effectiveness in lightening the skin in monotherapy became apparent, and today they are often included in lightening preparations.

There is still no consensus on the depigmenting effect of retinoids — inhibition of tyrosinase synthesis, disruption of melanosome transfer, and pigment dispersion in keratinocytes are assumed. Still, these effects are subtle and seem to be mediated. On the other hand, retinol has a considerable skin tone leveling effect and can be used in combination therapy for pigmentation. However, we should remember that retinoids induce the production of pro-inflammatory cytokines, cause irritation, and may directly stimulate hyperpigmentation. Besides, they are photosensitizers; that is, they increase skin sensitivity to the sun. Therefore, their use should always be accompanied by sunscreens and, preferably, anti-inflammatory products.

Dermatological preparations can include tretinoin, tazarotene, and adapalene. Tretinoin can irritate the skin, setting the stage for the development of post-inflammatory pigmentation. Adapalene and tazarotene can be used to treat post-inflammatory hyperpigmentation in patients with acne. A fourth-generation retinoid, tripharotene, received FDA approval in late 2019. According to the available studies, tripharotene has almost all the therapeutic properties of classical retinoids (anti-inflammatory, comedolytic, and depigmenting) but causes fewer unpleasant side effects, such as irritation and flaking. This beneficial effect is due to the selective binding of tripharotene only to retinoic acid receptors like RAR-y, which are expressed predominantly in epidermal cells and are virtually absent from dermal cells (Balak D.M.W., 2018). Retinol and its esters (retinyl acetate, retinaldehyde) are used in cosmetic products.

1.1.6. Whitening cosmetic formulations always contain a combination of ingredients aimed at different targets

The ideal whitening agent should:
- Lighten existing pigmentation
- Normalize melanin production and its transport from melanocytes to keratinocytes
- Eliminate the cause of pigmentation
- Be safe

None of the cosmetics on the market today has all these properties. However, many modern depigmenting agents act on several links of melanogenesis simultaneously, and their safety level is much higher than that of hydroquinone. Though not comparable yet, many of these products exhibit similar efficiency as hydroquinone. But their strength lies in the combination.

Thus, the development of an effective depigmenting agent is presently carried out in three main directions:
1. Searching for a safe depigmenting agent as an alternative to hydroquinone

2. Searching for successful combinations of depigmenting agents in such a way that they affect the greatest number of targets in the melanogenesis pathway
3. Finding successful combinations of depigmenting agents with "supporting" substances that lighten the skin by exfoliating and creating conditions for suppressing melanocyte activity

We touched on exfoliating ingredients in this section; next, we will talk about substances that create conditions conductive to the melanocyte activity reduction.

1.2. Sunscreens

As we said before, the use of sunscreens is compulsory during the treatment of pigment lesions because UV radiation is the main activator of melanin synthesis.

1.2.1. UV filters

UV filters are the main substances in any sunscreen. They are divided into two groups according to their mechanism of action (**Table III-1-2**):
- Physical UV filters reflect and scatter UV rays
- Chemical UV filters absorb UV rays and transform the absorbed energy into heat

The "strongest" **chemical UV filters** are synthesized organic substances (e.g., benzophenones, cinnamates, salicylates, camphor, and para-aminobenzoic acid derivatives). Substances of natural origin provide less effective UV protection — these are plant pigments that can absorb UV energy (e.g., caffeic acid). Natural UV filters are introduced into formulations as auxiliary ingredients to attract natural cosmetics supporters.

Physical UV filters (also called barrier filters) include micronized insoluble particles of titanium dioxide (Ti_2O) and zinc oxide (ZnO). They have an excellent safety record and protect the skin from a wide range of UV radiation. But there is one limitation here — the microparticles

Table III-1-2. UV filters: action, properties, representatives

CRITERIA	CHEMICAL UV FILTERS	PHYSICAL UV FILTERS
Chemical nature	Organic compounds	Inorganic particles (< 1 µm)
Mechanism of action	Absorb UV rays with subsequent release of heat (infrared radiation)	Reflect and scatter UV rays
Distribution in the skin	Across and within the *stratum corneum*	Across the *stratum corneum*
Penetration	Very low	No penetration
Benefits	• High level of security • Possibility to create combinations with minimal "working" concentrations and a wide protective spectrum • Good "cosmetic" effect • Good compatibility with other formulation components	• High level of security • UVA/B protection • Inertness against UV rays
Disadvantages	Potential phototoxicity due to phototransformation upon UV absorption (approved substances have successfully passed long-term safety tests, so the risks here are close to zero)	• The "whitewash" effect • Precipitation • Difficulties when combined with some other components of the formulation • Quite high "working" concentrations
UV filters approved for use in cosmetics in the EC: INCI* and brand names (in parentheses)		
UVA filters (400–315 nm)	• Avobenzone (Parsol 1789) • Bisdisulizole disodium (Neo Heliopan AP) • Diethylamino hydroxybenzoyl hexyl benzoate (Uvinul A Plus) • Ecamsule (Mexoryl SX)** • Methyl anthranilate	No available substances

Continued on p. 109

Continued on p. 109

CRITERIA	CHEMICAL UV FILTERS	PHYSICAL UV FILTERS
UVB filters (315–290 nm)	• 4-Aminobenzoic acid (PABA) • Cinoxate • Ethylhexyl triazone (Uvinul T 150) • Homosalate • 4-Methylbenzylidene camphor (Parsol 5000) • Octyl methoxycinnamate (Octinoxate) • Octyl salicylate (Octisalate) • Padimate O (Escalol 507) • Phenylbenzimidazole sulfonic acid (Ensulizole) • Polysilicone-15 (Parsol SLX) • Trolamine salicylate	No available substances
UVA/B filters	• Bemotrizinol (Tinosorb S) • Benzophenones 1–12 • Dioxybenzone • Drometrizole trisiloxane (Mexoryl XL)** • Iscotrizinol (Uvasorb HEB) • Octocrylene • Oxybenzone (Benzophenone-3) • Sulisobenzone	• Titanium dioxide • Zinc oxide • Cerium oxide/dioxide **Hybrid (chemical/ physical):** • Bisoctrizole (Tinosorb M)

* International Nomenclature of Cosmetic Ingredients

** The Mexoryl UV filters® SX and XL are patented by L'Oréal and are found only in their products.

stain the skin white. This so-called "whitening effect" can be combated by reducing the size of the particles, for example, to the nanoscale. However, this leads to another serious problem —under UV light, very small titanium dioxide particles become photocatalysts and can trigger chemical reactions between other ingredients in the preparation. To prevent this process from occurring, the surface of the particles is modified by applying a special polymer coating.

Cerium (Ce)-based UV filters — phosphates and oxides/dioxides — have also been developed. A comparison of the photoprotective properties of cerium oxide with titanium dioxide and zinc dioxide shows an even more pronounced filter efficacy. However, despite initial hopes of non-toxicity, cerium oxide nanoforms, like nanoforms of other physical filters, are also characterized by potent cytotoxicity and pro-oxidant activity (Miri A. et al., 2020). However, micronized forms of all these filters are currently considered the safest.

Hydroxyapatites are promising candidates for the role of a physical UV filter. By itself, tricalcium phosphate ($Ca_3(PO_4)_2$) does not absorb or reflect UV.

However, if zinc and manganese ions were added, the combined material would be an even more powerful UV filter than the alternatives based on Ti_2O and ZnO.

Silicone microparticles of 0.3–0.5 µm diameter also have UV filter properties. They reflect rays not only in the UV part but also in the visible portion of the spectrum. Due to recent studies on the possible negative effects of visible light on the skin, this property becomes interesting.

Plants, fungi, and bacteria also synthesize black pigments that protect them from excessive UV radiation. They are called **allomelanin** and are formed from diphenols and do not contain nitrogen. Allomelanin is now being studied for its possible use in sunscreen cosmetics, which is also a very promising direction.

Another interesting trend in sun protection is the use of photolyases, enzymes capable of repairing UV-derived CPD mutations. In nature, photolyases are naturally synthesized by bacteria, plants, and animals exposed to high levels of sun exposure; in humans, they are absent.

1.2.2. Protection against visible light

As for protection against visible light, the blue part of the spectrum, which can also lead to the development of pigmentation, it is only provided by reflecting or scattering light. Inorganic sunscreens, primarily iron oxide, but also titanium dioxide or zinc oxide, can help, since their reflectance spans from the UV to the visible part of the spectrum (Sondenheimer K., Krutmann J., 2018).

1.2.3. Safety

In addition to the issue with nanoscale forms of physical filters that we mentioned above, there are concerns about the photostability and safety of chemical filters. In early 2019, the U.S. FDA declared para-aminobenzoic acid (PABA) and trolamine salicylate unsafe for use in sunscreens. Benzophenone-3 and -4, avobenzone, and octocrylene have also been declared unsafe. They are allergens (in 2014, the American Contact Dermatitis Society named benzophenones allergens of the year), can irritate the skin, and some studies have tentatively demonstrated endocrine system effects (again, benzophenones seem to be implicated in this process). However, there is currently no reliable evidence that they can pose a systemic health risk in the quantities used in sunscreens.

Even though the authors of several recent studies have indeed recorded the ability of chemical filters to enter the bloodstream, they do not (Matta M.K. et al., 2019; Matta M.K. et al., 2020). It should be noted that these observations were based on the administration of very large amounts of sunscreen (2 mg/cm^2 on 75% of the body surface four times a day every two hours), which, in reality, is seldom applied. Moreover, just because UV filters are found in plasma this does not make them indiscriminately harmful to the body, nor does the fact that their concentration exceeds the 0.5 ng/ml limit make these ingredients unconditionally toxic. It is important to understand that **0.5 ng/ml is a conditional, probability-based concentration of a substance in the blood. Below this threshold, one can consider that no additional safety studies are required for the substance concerning its effect on carcinogenesis. Its detection in higher concentrations merely indicates the need to collect additional safety data** (Charalambides M. et al., 2020).

It should not be forgotten that risk is not a synonym for danger. Currently, no risks have been identified for the UV filters studied that would justify banning them, and they are all still approved for use in cosmetics worldwide. On the other hand, there is ample evidence that excessive exposure to the sun causes more than photoaging: the primary health risk is that UV radiation can cause skin cancer; sunburns from childhood are particularly dangerous. Sunscreens used according to the recommended guidelines are a reliable way to prevent skin cancer. Some prominent scientists who have studied the concentration of UV filters in the blood concur that, without further research, it is impossible to assess what absorption level of UV filters can be considered safe. The need for such studies does not yet suggest that using sunscreen cosmetics is a health hazard.

Commercial UV filters are inevitably developed based on a compromise among efficacy, safety, and consumer appeal. For example, product effectiveness can be increased if there are many filters in the formula, even in small amounts. Such a formula will be safer than a product with a "strong" but potentially allergenic filter, although this is an expensive way to go. In terms of manufacturing, topical sunscreens are probably among the most difficult categories of cosmetics, requiring considerable experience and a good science and technology base. There are many nuances to consider when creating a sunscreen formulation, which we will discuss below.

1.2.4. Requirements for sunscreen products

A layer of sunscreen remains in contact with the skin for an extended period. Unlike skincare products, the use of which implies an active effect on the skin, the main task of sunscreen, as its name suggests, is **protection** — the reflection of aggressive external factors, UV radiation in particular.

Accordingly, sunscreen formulation design is based on seven basic requirements:

1. **Good skin tolerance.** The aim here is to allow the user to apply the product and forget about it. Even if the skin is sensitive, it should not notice the protective layer covering it, much less react to it with irritation or discomfort.
2. **Good consumer qualities.** The only acceptable feeling one can have after applying sunscreen is the sense of comfort from well-moisturized and softened skin. Its use should also instill confidence that the skin is protected. The product should not form a heavy, greasy layer, be sticky, collect dust, or produce the "whitewash effect" (typical for earlier sunscreen formulations based on titanium dioxide and zinc oxide — physical

UV filters that reflect UV rays), or make the skin appear lacquered. It is best if the layer is not visible at all.

3. **Non-toxicity.** Sunscreens are usually applied to large areas of the body, and the risk of percutaneous absorption into the body of a particular substance in a dose greater than the permissible amount to preclude toxicity should be minimal. Only compounds that do not pass through the *stratum corneum* are allowed for use in cosmetics (if a substance can pass through undamaged barrier structures on its own, then it must be classified as a drug). Modern UV filters "work" **only** on the skin surface, aiming to prevent the penetration of UV rays.

4. **Photostability.** The issue of sunscreen safety and efficacy is closely related to the reactivity of their ingredients with photons. Likewise, spontaneous photochemical reactions between individual components can start under the influence of solar radiation, resulting in "unplanned" substances in the product that are potentially dangerous to the skin. Another option is photo-induced changes in the substances (including those UV filters), which can become toxic and cause unwanted skin reactions (e.g., photodermatitis). Due to their instability and phototoxicity, many substances successfully tested for their absorption efficacy have subsequently not been approved.

5. **UV absorption spectrum.** This is the most important characteristic and indicates the ability to protect the skin from photodamage in general and photodermatitis in particular. The first drugs that were introduced to the market for this purpose aimed to prevent sunburn and erythema development in response to UVB radiation. Over the last fifteen years, the skin's reaction to UVA radiation has been actively studied. The role of UVA radiation in suppressing skin immunity as well as in the development of chronic photodamage is no longer questioned by anyone. That's why both UVA and UVB filters are included in formulations. The reality is that the selection of UVB filters approved for use is much wider than UVA filters. The difficulty with chemical UVA filters stems from the fact that the better a substance absorbs rays in the long-wavelength UVA part of the spectrum, the more yellow its color becomes and the less stable it is in the light.

6. **Water resistance.** The protective layer must repel water; otherwise, it will quickly wash off, leaving the skin unprotected. We usually apply sunscreen when we go to the beach. This means that the water we immerse ourselves in and the sweat naturally released in the heat should not compromise the sunscreen coverage. Water resistance is ensured by specially selected components of the product's base, where UV filters are "immersed."

7. **Claimed photoprotection.** This is a very subtle aspect, although it is the first thing people pay attention to when choosing a product. There was a time when the sun protection factor was supposed to be maximal, and manufacturing companies were competing to see who would produce the most reliable sunblock with the highest SPF. The higher the number, the more enticing the product looked in the eyes of consumers. There were even products with SPF 100+ on the market! However, the higher SPF number does not provide the same multiplicity of photoprotection. For example, SPF 2 blocks 50% of UVB, SPF 4 — 75%, SPF 15 — 93.3%, SPF 30 — 96.7%, SPF 50 — 98%, and SPF 100 — 99%. In other words, there is only one extra percentage behind the flashy number "100" compared to SPF 50. On the other hand, this degree of UV blockage is only noted if the consumer uses the sunscreen application mode recommended by the manufacturer. We'll talk about that below.

Still, it is the manufacturer's responsibility to ensure that the promised photoprotection is provided. This requires, first and foremost, clear criteria and quantitative indicators based on which developers create, experts evaluate, and consumers choose the product.

UVB protection: SPF — sun protection factor

SPF is the most commonly used parameter to show how effectively a product protects the skin from sunburn and erythema. It is based on an estimate of the minimal erythema dose (MED) — the dose of UV radiation that would cause erythema 24 hours after insolation.

The MED of the unprotected skin area is measured and compared with the MED of the skin to which the product is applied to assess how effectively the product under test protects the skin from burns. The SPF value indicates how many times the MED of protected skin is greater than that of unprotected skin. Since sunburns are caused by UVB rays, SPF indicates only the degree of protection from UVB radiation.

The MED depends on the skin phototype. For example, for phototype I, the safe tanning time when the UV index is equal to 6 will be 20 minutes, and for a person with III phototype — 40 minutes. Such difference relates to the fact that constitutive melanin of non-tanned people of different phototypes ensures different degrees of photoprotection. For example, the intrinsic epidermal melanin of people with skin phototype VI gives UVB protection equivalent to SPF 13.4, compared to 3.4 for fair skin. In addition, the epidermis of dark skin transmits 7.4% of UVB radiation compared to 29.4% for light skin, and 17.5% compared to 55.5% of UVA rays, respectively (Kaidbey K.H. et al., 1979). These numbers increase with the appearance of tanning and are characteristic of non-tanned skin. A tan gives an average of +3 SPF units.

The higher the product's SPF value, the stronger the protection. The lighter the skin, the higher the SPF needed for adequate protection. For example, if the skin is very light and a person can stay in the sun without blushing for only 5 minutes on average, applying SPF 8 could theoretically prolong the pleasure by 8 times, i.e., 5 minutes × 8 = 40 minutes.

It is not that simple, though. In reality, the SPF value depends on many factors: phototype, amount of the applied preparation, and external conditions of "operation" (e.g., intensity of UV radiation, contact with water, friction against sand). In particular, the SPF determination requires that the preparation being tested is applied in 2 mg/cm^2. But the average person uses only about 0.5 mg/cm^2. As a result, the promised sun protection is at least four times weaker. When applying a product with SPF 50 in such a "low-quality" way, the actual safe tanning time increases by 12.5 times, not 50.

Therefore, regulatory authorities in the EU and the USA are now changing their approach to maximum SPF values. For example, while the recommended upper limit of SPF was recently 50+, in February 2019, the FDA proposed raising this number to 60+. In South America, sunscreens are graded SPF from 6 to 99 (Krutmann J. et al., 2020). All of this suggests that SPF is not a guarantee but only a guideline for product selection.

Today the SPF indicator can also be found on cosmetic products of other categories (e.g., skincare products, makeup foundation, decorative powder, lipstick). Any non-washable product on the skin during the day can contain a certain amount of UV filters, which is the basis for claiming its sun protection properties.

In contrast to the first care products characterized by a low level of SPF (10–15), today, many popular brands have begun to produce creams with SPF in the 30–50 range, which is equivalent to the SPF of traditional sunscreens. Since this is the case, it would be logical to assume that we can also talk about an equivalent level of real protection that these creams provide. However, a recent study comparing the effectiveness of the UV protection provided by applying traditional sunscreens and a moisturizer with a similar SPF level demonstrated that this was not the case (Lourenco E.A.J. et al., 2019).

Volunteers were photographed in UVA light with a UV-sensitive camera — this shooting mode helps to capture areas that are impervious to UV light ("dark" areas in photos). The same areas with insufficient protection pass UV light and look lighter. The brighter the area, the lower the UV protection in these areas. Blind evaluation of the photographs showed that the participants' faces looked darker after applying sunscreen than after using moisturizer — i.e., in the latter case, protection was lower. Subsequent recalculation of the results with correction for additional chemical filters revealed an even greater difference in the values obtained.

However, as the authors found out, it was not the moisturizer itself (the tests showed that it has even higher UV-filtering properties than the sunscreen). The problem was in the quality of product application. For example, the moisturizer had significantly worse facial area coverage — participants missed an average of 16.6% of the skin surface, compared to 11.1% for the sunscreen. The eyelids were primarily affected. This area was missed 20.9% of the time when moisturizers were applied and 14% of the time when sunscreen was used. Interestingly, all participants were confident that both products were applied to the face "without skipping."

The authors attribute the reason for these results primarily to the habit of using moisturizers in much smaller quantities than sunscreens. Interestingly, the percentage of missed areas was higher for women than for men. Another possible reason, according to the authors, could be the different viscosity of the products presented, due to which achieving even moisturizer distribution was somewhat more difficult than the sunscreen application.

An important point emphasized by specialists is the tendency to repeatedly miss the same areas, in contrast to the more general problem of incomplete coverage of the entire surface of the face. At the same time, according to the available evidence, the eyelid area is one of the most frequent localizations of skin cancer. Recent research further shows that the sunscreen under-application is also a major problem, leading to the false sense of protection when in the sun.

UVA protection: PPD — persistent pigment darkening reaction

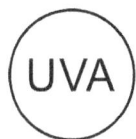

UVA radiation does not cause erythema, but, as we said, it induces the appearance of immediate pigmentation with a subsequent transformation into persistent pigmentation. Using its evaluation, one can obtain data on the effectiveness of the sunscreen against UVA rays. The evaluation is performed two hours after the irradiation (which is sufficient for the appearance of stable pigmentation). Darkening due to melanin photooxidation is characteristic of all skin types except phototype I.

Japanese scientists developed the PPD method and then introduced it into the cosmetics industry with the support of several companies, including L'Oréal. Like SPF, PPD indicates how much better the skin is protected by the tested product. Theoretically, a product with a PPD of 10 could prolong sun exposure by 10 times without the appearance of a tan.

The PPD method is now officially included by Colipa International in the list of required tests that every new sunscreen product must pass before it enters the market. According to the European cosmetics legislation, every sunscreen must provide minimal protection against

UVA rays. If a product's PPD is more than 1/3 of its SPF, the product is eligible for a special label.

At the same time, Asian manufacturers use the "RA" label with different numbers of "+" signs to show the effectiveness of UVA protection.

DNA PF — DNA protection factor

This figure shows how effectively the sunscreen prevents the formation of pyrimidine dimers in the DNA molecule. According to experimental data, for a product with an SPF of 15, the measured DNA PF is about 50, and products with an SPF of 4 still protect the cellular genetic apparatus well enough (DNA PF of about 10). According to van Praag M.C. et al. (1993), SPF 10 provides excellent DNA protection.

IPF — immune protection factor

The immune protection factor (IPF) suggested by Barnetson is independent of the SPF value and is only determined by the spectral characteristics of the UV filter (Damian D.L. et al., 1999). Broad-spectrum UV filters provide the best protection of skin immunity from UV radiation. Since the ability of sunscreens to prevent immunosuppression correlates with their ability to prevent UV-induced carcinogenesis, it has been proposed to introduce IPF evaluation as a mandatory efficacy test. While such tests would certainly be valuable, at present, this important information is yet to be included on the labels of commercial sunscreens.

1.2.5. Development of sunscreen formulation

How do you make sure the sunscreen formula meets the requirements listed above? There are several ways to do this.

Combination of several UV filters — maximum protection and minimum concentration

At first glance, increasing the concentration of UV filters is enough to increase the SPF and PPD. However, this approach is unacceptable because it contradicts the safety requirements. In addition, there are technical limitations due to the deterioration of the properties consumers expect from the product. Therefore, the only correct way is to include in the formulation a combination of UV filters with different absorption properties (targeting UVA and/or UVB) and, preferably, different solubility (water- and oil-soluble). First, reliance on this strategy reduces the total concentration of UV filters in the system — including "strong" filters with a controversial safety profile. Second, the combined use of UV filters expands the range of protection. Another reason is that UV filters have varying degrees of photostability. By combining several substances, we make the system more resistant to light.

Product base — a guarantee of stability and good textural properties

Optimizing the spectral and chemical characteristics of the UV filter combination is important, but it is not the only point. Let's imagine a very real situation: the product stratifies or precipitates during storage. In this case, the distribution of UV filters in its volume becomes heterogeneous, which means that when the product is applied to the skin, some areas have more UV filters, and some have less.

Its base largely determines the sun protection properties of the product. It ensures an even distribution of UV filters over the surface, easy application, and the ability to create a uniform coating, water resistance, and good adhesion to the skin. The base should not contain substances that oxidize or decompose quickly in light (e.g., unsaturated fatty acids). Silicones (organosilicon compounds) are superior to their organic counterparts in this regard — modern sunscreens are silicone-based (mostly high-molecular-weight silicone oils). As for organic compounds, hydrocarbons in small quantities are acceptable (e.g., mineral oil, paraffin, liquid vaseline) — they are good solvents, but their consumer properties are inferior to silicone oils. Therefore, as a rule, the base combines organic and silicone oils in which oil-soluble chemical UV filters are dissolved or microparticles (zinc oxide, titanium dioxide) are dispersed.

Among UV filters, there are water-soluble substances, and an aqueous phase is required for their inclusion in the formulation. However, preparations with a high water content are unsuitable for photoprotection because they wash off quickly. Thus, the only option when using water-soluble UV filters is to include them in an emulsion system consisting of two phases — water and oil. This requires emulsifiers — substances without which an emulsion cannot exist. Emulsifiers have been the subject of a great deal of criticism from dermatologists, as they represent a real threat to the lipid barrier of the *stratum corneum*. The cosmetics industry has been searching for dermatologically friendly emulsifiers, and we must say there has been great success. However, reducing the concentration of emulsifiers is one of the most important tasks, especially when we are talking about a product that will be in contact with the skin for a long time, especially under stressful implied from insolation conditions.

Substances with additional valuable properties

Sunscreen formulations include substances that give the finished product additional properties — for example, moisturizing components, anti-inflammatory agents, antioxidants (usually oil-soluble vitamin E), and even immunomodulators (yeast polysaccharides, chitosan). However, the main thing here is not to overdo it. There is a general rule: the higher the degree of photoprotection, the lower the amount of additional "active" substances in the formulation. There is a reason for that: sunscreen with a high photoprotection factor should restrain the "pressure" of UV radiation for a long time, meaning anything that can potentially increase the skin's photosensitivity should be avoided. Fragrances and colorants are also highly undesirable.

Another nuance is the introduction of anti-inflammatory agents into sunscreens. Since the only sign of pronounced photodamage to the skin is the appearance of erythema, and they "take it away," there are concerns that their inclusion in the formulation may give people a false sense of security. "Since my skin hasn't reddened yet, that means the sunscreen is working, and I'm protected," when that may not be true.

On the other hand, the use of photostable antioxidants in the formula is welcome. Not only do they not reduce the product's sun protection ability, but they also increase the level of skin protection from free radicals formed under the influence of UV radiation. Vitamin E directly protects cells from forming "dark" CPD (Delinasios G.J. et al., 2018).

1.2.6. How to choose the correct sunscreen

Surveys conducted among modern consumers show that those who are aware of the damage caused by the sun prefer products with maximum photoprotective effect. How sensible is this?

Recall that most of us have skin that can protect itself and adapt to the daily dose of UV light. The skin begins to produce and accumulate a natural UV filter, the melanin pigment, the thickness of the *stratum corneum* increases, and other protective mechanisms are mobilized, including the antioxidant system and immune cells. All these adaptation processes triggered in response to a sub-threshold stressor are beneficial and make the skin more resilient. Now imagine that your skin was constantly covered in a layer of "sun blocker," and then suddenly, for some reason, it was left uncovered and exposed to the sun's rays. Unprepared skin is damaged much faster. So, a person who applies sunscreen daily and spends much time in the sun is probably at a much higher risk than someone who doesn't apply it at all but reasonably avoids the sun.

Let's also remember that vitamin D is synthesized in the skin under UV light, and its deficit in the body leads to osteoporosis, rickets, and skin problems. This fact should not be forgotten by residents of northern countries, which are not blessed with too many sunny days. But if a pale-faced northerner decides to go to the south, diligent sunscreen application will be mandatory because his skin is poorly adapted to the sun!

Sunscreen use is also obligatory in any pigmentation treatment program.

When choosing a sunscreen, you should first determine its objectives. If it is just for daily prevention means, choosing a suitable day cream and powder with UV filters is sufficient. If you are going to nature, you should be guided by climatic and geographical features: consider the season, the altitude above sea level, and the presence of reflective surfaces (water, sand, snow). As a rule, the higher the estimated dose of UV exposure, the stronger the photoprotection must be. Of course, the skin's pigment production capacity (phototype) must also be considered.

Based on the insolation intensity, we can determine the UV index, which characterizes the intensity of UV radiation in a specific geographic

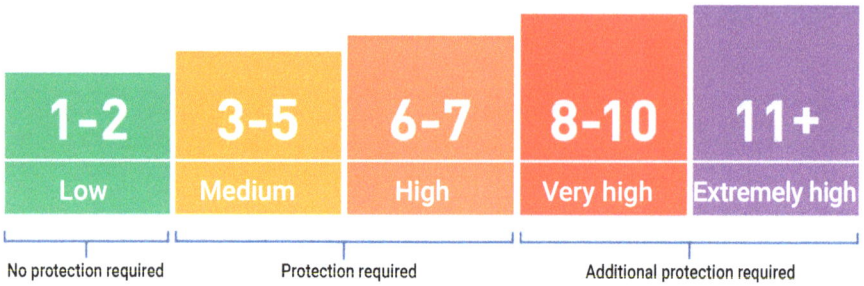

Figure III-1-3. Recommendations for the use of sunscreens based on UV index values

location at a specific time. Knowing the UV index, it is possible to individually select sunscreens of different strengths. Many online resources and apps display the UV index according to geolocation. In general, the use of photoprotectors is considered necessary if the UV index exceeds 3 (**Fig. III-1-3**).

The time you can spend in the sun without harming your skin can also be determined visually using a graph (**Fig. III-1-4**) (Sánchez-Pérez J.F. et al., 2019). If the time spent in the sun exceeds the duration deemed "safe," sunscreen should be used.

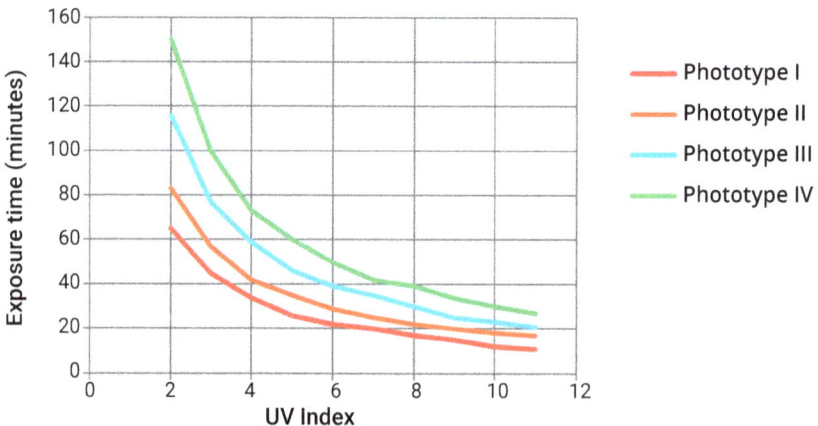

Figure III-1-4. Relationship between exposure time for the appearance of first-degree sunburn and UV index for several skin phototypes and 1 Minimal Erythema Dose (MED) according to DIN-5050 for clear sky days (adapted from Sánchez-Pérez J.F. et al., 2019)

Another important point is that the product must protect against a wide range of UV rays. However, most modern sunscreen formulas take this requirement into account.

Still, in some cases, blocking UV rays from reaching the skin completely is necessary, even if the person has no pigmentation problems. For example, this would be essential after a traumatic aesthetic procedure (peeling, dermabrasion, mesotherapy), surgery, or burns — until the skin regains its barrier properties and the inflammation subsides, it cannot be exposed to UV stress. Likewise, a person taking photosensitizing medications must avoid direct light.

In **Table III-1-3**, the most common photosensitizers capable of causing phototoxic (associated with direct cell damage and accelerating sunburn) and photoallergic (immune events like dermatitis) reactions are

Table III-1-3. Photosensitizing drugs

GROUP	COMPOUND	PHOTOTOXIC REACTION	PHOTOALLERGIC REACTION
Antibiotics	Tetracyclines (doxycycline, tetracycline)	Yes	No
	Fluoroquinolones (ciprofloxacin, ofloxacin, levofloxacin)	Yes	No
	Sulfonamides	Yes	No
Antiviral	Acyclovir	No	Yes
Nonsteroidal anti-inflammatory drugs	Ibuprofen	Yes	No
	Ketoprofen	Yes	Yes
	Naproxen	Yes	No
	Celecoxib	No	Yes
Hormonal medications	Hydrocortisone	No	Yes
Diuretics	Furosemide	Yes	No
	Bumetanide	No	No
	Hydrochlorthiazide	Yes	No
Retinoids	Isotretinoin	Yes	No
	Acitretin	Yes	No

Continued on p. 124

GROUP	COMPOUND	PHOTOTOXIC REACTION	PHOTOALLERGIC REACTION
Hypoglyce-mic drugs	Sulfonylureas (glipizide, glyburide)	No	Yes
HMG-CoA reductase inhibitors	Statins (atorvastatin, fluvas-tatin, lovastatin, pravastatin, simvastatin)	Yes	Yes
Epidermal growth fac-tor inhibi-tors	Cetuximab, panitumu-mumab, erlotinib, gefitinib, lapatinib, vandetanib	Yes	Yes
Antipsy-chotic drugs	Phenothiazines (chlor-promazine, fluphenazine, perazine, perphenazine, thioridazine)	Yes	Yes
	Thioxanthenes (chlorprotix-ene, thiotixene)	Yes	No
Antifungal	Terbinafine	No	No
	Itraconazole	Yes	Yes
	Voriconazole	Yes	No
	Griseofulvin	Yes	Yes
Different groups	Para-aminobenzoic acid	Yes	Yes
	5-Fluorouracil	Yes	Yes
	Paclitaxel	Yes	No
	Amiodarone	Yes	No
	Diltiazem	Yes	No
	Quinidine	Yes	Yes
	Hydroxychloroquine	No	No
	Nifedipine	Yes	No
	Enalapril	No	No
	Dapson	No	Yes
	Oral contraceptives	No	Yes

Continued on p. 125

GROUP	COMPOUND	PHOTOTOXIC REACTION	PHOTOALLERGIC REACTION
Alpha hy-droxy acids	Glycolic acid	Yes (in high concentra-tion)	Yes
Sunscreens	Para-aminobenzoic acid	No	Yes
	Cinnamic acid esters (cinnamates)	No	Yes
	Benzophenones	No	Yes
	Salicylates	No	Yes
Fragrances	Ambrettolide	No	Yes
	6-Methylcoumarin	No	Yes
	Essential oils (bergamot, cumin, ginger, lemon, lime, mandarin, orange, and verbena)	No (yes for bergamot)	Yes

listed. Information about using these medications (and even perfume) is important to obtain while collecting the patient's medical history. In all these situations, the patient must use products with the maximum protection factor, ideally those based on physical UV filters — titanium dioxide and zinc oxide.

1.3. Antioxidants

Antioxidants are natural or synthetic substances capable of slowing down oxidation. They are considered mainly in the context of the oxidation of organic compounds.

An antioxidant can lower the amount of ROS and free radicals and prevent the development of radical chain reactions. Usually, an antioxidant sacrifices itself, i.e., it reacts with ROS, turning them into chemically stable and inactive molecules. The antioxidant becomes a free radical but chemically much less active. In this form, it is not dangerous

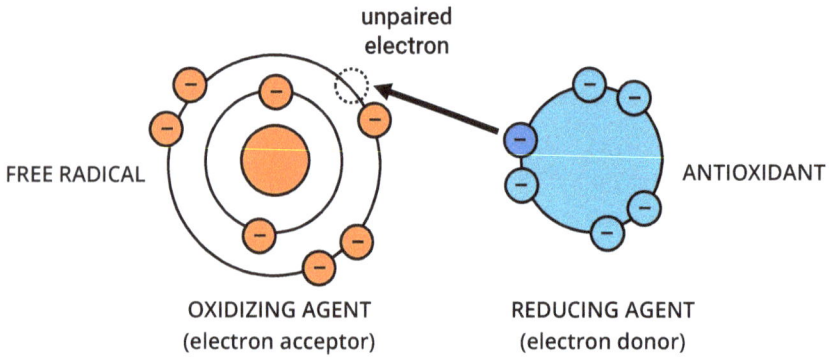

In a reduction-oxidation (redox) reaction, an electron transfer occurs from the reducing agent (electron donor) to the oxidizing agent (electron acceptor)

unpaired electron

FREE RADICAL

ANTIOXIDANT

OXIDIZING AGENT
(electron acceptor)

REDUCING AGENT
(electron donor)

Figure III-1-5. The antioxidant gives its electron to the free radical, thereby reducing it to a stable form

to the environment, but it is also non-functional — until it is restored to its active state (**Fig. III-1-5**). Thus, **the antioxidant molecule, once reacted, loses its power**.

One substance is not enough for antioxidant protection to work smoothly and constantly. Evolution has developed a multi-level antioxidant system in the body, with different parts of the system supporting and restoring each other:

- **Enzymatic antioxidants** — superoxide dismutase, catalase, peroxidase, glutathione reductase, and reduced glutathione
- **Macromolecular non-enzymatic antioxidants** — transferrin (iron carrier protein) and other serum proteins capable of binding iron ions* (ceruloplasmin, haptoglobin, hemopexin)
- **Low-molecular-weight antioxidants** — female sex hormones, thyroxine, flavonoids, steroid hormones, vitamins C, E, P, ubiquinone, carnosine, low-molecular-weight sulfur-containing compounds, and selenium

_____

* Iron ions are related to pro-oxidants — compounds that trigger free-radical chain reactions

Our body synthesizes most antioxidants on its own, replenishing them as needed. However, some of them (e.g., vitamin C, flavonoids, selenium) come from food. Antioxidants vary in potency, specificity (i.e., "targets"), and mechanisms of action. In addition, some are oil-soluble and "work" in the lipid phase (in membranes, preventing lipid peroxidation). In contrast, others are water-soluble and protect water-soluble compounds from free-radical attacks.

The greatest antioxidant effect is achieved when antioxidants act in pairs or groups. After giving its electron to a free radical, the antioxidant is oxidized and inactivated. To make it work again, it must be restored. For example, glutathione restores vitamin C, and vitamin C restores vitamin E.

1.3.1. Natural antioxidants in cosmetic products

The most popular cosmetic antioxidants include the following substances.

Vitamin E (tocopherol)

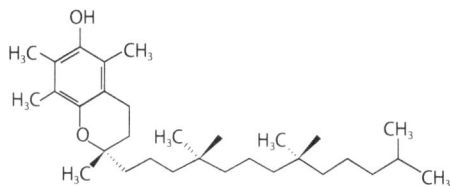

It includes eight oil-soluble substances, such as α- and β-tocopherols and tocotrienols. In skincare, α-tocopherol is more commonly used. Vitamin E is the body's main oil-soluble antioxidant and is particularly effective in preventing lipid peroxidation. For this reason, vitamin E is considered the main protector of cell membranes and the skin's lipid barrier. Its ability to prevent UV-induced skin damage and reduce inflammation has been well documented. Vitamin E is oxidized by interaction with free radicals and loses its activity. In the cell, vitamin E is regenerated by vitamin C. Since vitamin C is water-soluble and vitamin E is oil-soluble, these two substances must meet at the cell membrane's border.

Vitamin C (L-ascorbic acid)

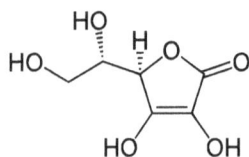

Vitamin C is the main water-soluble antioxidant of cells. Because vitamin C is easily destroyed, its derivatives, which have greater stability (ascorbyl palmitate, sodium ascorbyl phosphate), are often used in cosmetics instead of ascorbic acid. In addition, as we mentioned above, it has depigmenting activity.

β-Carotene

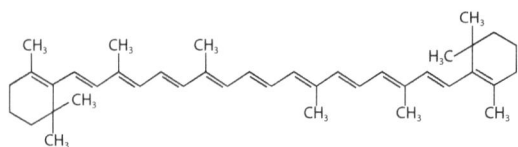

Orange pigment in plants. It is especially plentiful in carrots, yams, pumpkins, and sea buckthorn. β-Carotene is a tetraterpene and differs from other carotenoids by the presence of two beta rings on its molecule. It specializes in neutralizing singlet oxygen. This molecule is the first free oxygen radical created in the skin when exposed to UV radiation. If there is enough β-carotene in the skin, reactions involving free radicals are inhibited in their initial stages.

α-Lipoic acid (thioctic acid)

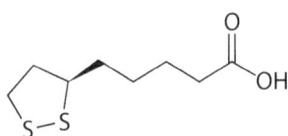

Lipoic acid is a powerful natural antioxidant that can both fight ROS on its own and increase the skin's antioxidant potential by restoring vitamins E and C expended in fighting free radicals. It slows down aging in the mitochondria, the cell's energy station. It is oil-soluble, so it easily passes through the *stratum corneum*.

Coenzyme Q_{10} (ubiquinone)

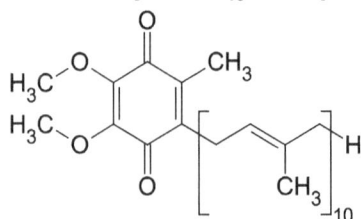

Ubiquinone is found in the membranes of all living cells, but its content is particularly high in the membranes of mitochondria. There is a good reason for this. The fact that this substance is necessary for the normal course of an important reaction, during which ATP, a molecule that is an energy carrier in living cells, is formed. This reaction is carried out on the membrane of the mitochondria. Coenzyme Q_{10} acts as an antioxidant not only in mitochondria but also in biological membranes and blood plasma. Moreover, its antioxidant effect is related to the direct interception of free radicals. Coenzyme Q_{10} also restores vitamin E, and due to its lipophilicity, it does so better than the well-known tocopherol-reducing agent ascorbic acid.

Antioxidant herbal compositions

It is not uncommon for antioxidants to be found in plant extract formulations. The following extracts are the richest in antioxidants.

Seaside pine (*Pinus pinaster*) **bark extract**, native to France, is enriched with proanthocyanins, substances comprising polymer chains of several flavonoids, such as catechin. It is taken orally as a dietary supplement (pycnogenol), but the extract can be included in a cosmetic product.

Green tea extract is obtained from the *Camellia sinensis* plant. Green tea was first cultivated in South Asia over 4,000 years ago. Different types of tea (white, yellow, green, black, and oolong) are produced by varying the drying methods and fermenting the tea leaves. Green tea contains catechins — the polyphenolic compounds that belong to the class of monomeric flavanols. The main catechins in green tea are epigallocatechin, epicatechin-3-gallate, and epicatechin. Green tea extract protects skin from UV damage by reducing the production of hydrogen peroxide, nitric oxide, and lipid peroxides, as well as by restoring the activity of antioxidant enzymes such as superoxide dismutase. In addition, green tea has been found to inhibit inflammation and stimulate skin cell division and collagen production.

Açai berry extract is obtained from the fruits of the açai palm (*Euterpe oleracea*) growing in the Amazon rainforest. They have long been used in traditional medicine to improve health, replenish strength, and restore the beauty of the skin and hair.

Today, the açai berry is considered the richest source of antioxidants, surpassing all other edible fruits. The açai palm fruit contains a complex antioxidant cocktail of 14 active substances at very low concentrations. Some antioxidants are "fast" and instantly neutralize destructive free radicals, while others are "slow" and can pass into cells unchanged and protect them from damage. Cold-pressed açai berry seed oil is a rich source of essential omega-3 and omega-6 fatty acids, vitamins, and antioxidants.

Polypodium leucotomos fern extract is a fern species native to the tropics and subtropics of eastern North and South America. The plant has been used in traditional Central American medicine for many ailments. *P. leucotomos* is a powerful antioxidant due to its high content of phenolic components. Its extract contains ferulic acid, which we spoke about when discussing depigmenting agents, as well as other phenolic acids (caffeic, vanillic, coumaric, chlorogenic, 3,4-dihydroxybenzoic, and others) and flavonoids. These plant pigments have antioxidant, anti-inflammatory, and antitumor properties. *P. leucotomos* fern extract prevents pro-inflammatory mechanisms underlying UV damage, including lipid peroxidation and ROS formation, reduces UV damage to DNA, stimulates the expression of anti-oncogene p53 and its activation, reduces MMP production and activates collagen synthesis, reduces inflammation severity and vasodilation, and inhibits the immunosuppressive effect of UV radiation within the skin (Parrado C. et al., 2016).

1.3.2. The art of antioxidant formulation

First, several antioxidants must be present in the drug. This is paramount because, after the reaction between the free radical and the antioxidant, the latter loses its activity. If there is only one antioxidant compound (even if in a high concentration), its active resource is very soon exhausted because there is no means of restoring it. In addition, after interacting with a free radical, the antioxidant itself becomes a free radical, albeit a very weak one. However, if the antioxidant concentration is high enough, a significant amount of weak free radicals accumulates in the product over time, and the drug may turn into its opposite, i.e., it intensifies skin damage.

Most cosmetic products contain both aqueous and oily phases, so both water- and oil-soluble antioxidants must be included in their formulation.

Antioxidants' lipophilic or hydrophilic nature affects their distribution in the skin and determines their access to free radicals.

Some ingredients in cosmetic formulations can interact with the active components and reduce their activity. It is also important to consider the activity of antioxidants and their long-term stability in finished formulations (**Table III-1-4**).

Table III-1-4. Information to consider when designing antioxidant formulations

BIOLOGICAL AND CHEMICAL CHARACTERISTICS	CONCLUSION
Free radicals are reactive molecules with lifetimes ranging from nano- to milliseconds.	The antioxidant must react very quickly with the ROS to "intercept" and neutralize them.
Most antioxidants neutralize free radicals through chemical reactions. Sometimes the reaction products are relatively stable radicals; for example, tocopherol, ascorbic acid, and quinones.	Intermediate radicals should also be neutralized to prevent the development of a chain reaction, which can also exacerbate the damage caused by ROS.
The antioxidant's ability to act as a reducing agent is determined by whether it is in an oxidized or reduced form. The reducing potential must be high enough for antioxidants to be able to reduce ROS.	In the formulation, it is necessary to include several antioxidants forming a self-repairing system. Such antioxidant systems exist in nature. These are, for example, plant bioflavonoids, which are characterized by the existence of many forms differing in their reducing potential.
The lipophilic or hydrophilic nature of antioxidants affects their distribution in the skin, and their accessibility to ROS.	Water- and oil-soluble antioxidants must be present in the formulation.
Some ingredients in cosmetic formulations can interact with active components and decrease their activity.	It is important to determine the antioxidant power and long-term stability in finished formulations.

Several antioxidants have a brightening and depigmenting effect. These include ascorbic acid and its more stable derivative ascorbyl magnesium phosphate, α-lipoic acid, melatonin, green tea extract, licorice, ginkgo, shiitake mushroom, and, of course, resveratrol and ferulic acid, which we discussed in the section on whitening agents. It is essential to note that ferulic acid is not only a powerful antioxidant but also stabilizes and enhances the activity of its "colleagues," particularly vitamins C and E, doubling their photoprotective ability.

Meanwhile, some experts say that the inclusion of antioxidants and depigmenting agents in the formulation can reduce the latter's effectiveness because the mechanism of action of some depigmenting compounds (mostly with a toxic effect) is based precisely on the generation of ROS in the skin. However, many modern drugs work in other ways. Regardless, it is useful to include antioxidant formulations in a cosmetic depigmentation program to reduce irritation and inflammation that can accompany the use of depigmentation products.

1.3.3. Selection algorithm for antioxidant skincare products

Unfortunately, not all cosmetic products on the market are effective. How can a consumer with no understanding of the technological process of antioxidant product manufacturing and no special training in medicine or biology figure out what is worth trying and what will almost certainly fall short of expectations? Let's give some general recommendations to help you in the antioxidant selection.

Antioxidant composition (primary antioxidant protection)

Most cosmetics contain aqueous and oily phases, so water- and oil-soluble antioxidants should be included in their formulation. The following antioxidants are most frequently found in skincare products:

- **Oil-soluble** — α-tocopherol (vitamin E) and its esters (tocopheryl acetate, tocopheryl palmitate), ubiquinone (vitamin Q_{10}), carotenoids (plant compounds: β-carotene, lutein, zeaxanthin, lycopene), ascorbyl palmitate (ester of vitamin C and palmitic fatty acid)

- **Water-soluble** — ascorbic acid (vitamin C) and its derivatives (magnesium ascorbyl phosphate, sodium ascorbyl phosphate), plant polyphenols (e.g., flavonoids), carnosine (dipeptide), sulfur-containing compounds (glutathione, cysteine, methionine), cinnamic acids (coumaric, caffeic, ferulic)

Often, antioxidants are included in the formulation as a part of plant extracts. There is a rationale for this since there are several antioxidant compounds present in natural mixtures, "selected" based on their redox potential* and in proportions optimal in terms of the system's ability to self-repair. Aqueous and oil extracts of the same plant differ in their composition, including antioxidant components. The antioxidant systems of oils are represented mainly by tocopherols and carotenoids, while phenolic compounds represent the aqueous extracts (e.g., polyphenols, cinnamic acids).

Antioxidants, individually and in natural mixtures, differ in their **antioxidant power** (**Fig. III-1-6**). The strongest oil-soluble antioxidant is α-tocopherol; among the water-soluble antioxidants is caffeic acid. Among vegetable oils, amaranth oil is considered one of the "strongest" in terms of antioxidant activity, while rosehip oil is slightly weaker. Among the aqueous extracts, the extracts of grape seed and maritime pine bark (commercial name — pycnogenol) are particularly noteworthy (they are rich in bioflavonoids), as well as the ink nut extract enriched with tannins.

However, the assessment of antioxidant power is always performed under *in vitro* conditions, i.e., outside the body, and only involves a single compound, without considering its interactions with other substances with which it is combined *in vivo*. Therefore, "antioxidant power" is certainly interesting as a comparative benchmark, but cannot be completely transferred to an extract or a ready-made cosmetic product.

_____

* Redox potential is a measure of a chemical's ability to attach electrons (reduction–oxidation reactions).

COMPOUND	ANTIOXIDANT POWER, AU	RELAXATION TIME, min
Water-soluble antioxidants		
L-ascorbic acid (vitamin C)	1,000,000	0.24
Caffeic acid	**2,032,910**	**0.159**
Aspalathin	**1,531,000**	**0.22**
Ellagic acid	**1,352,000**	**0.60**
Dihydroquercetin	**1,030,000**	**0.23**
Grape seed extract	357,000–930,000	0.95–0.81
Rooibos leaf extract	90,000–715,000	0.33–0.79
Tee leaf extract	375,946	0.705
Rosemary leaf extract	243,500	0.79
Ink nuts extract	739,340	0.61
Hops extract	109,660	1.01
Ginger extract	98,700	0.73
L-glutathione (reduced)	2,938	4.8
L-carnosine	224	3.82
Oil-soluble antioxidants		
Tocopherol (vitamin E)	404,000	0.33
Tocopherol acetate	0	—
Amaranth oil	730	0.31
Rosehip oil	457	0.794
Borage oil	295	1.08
Wheat bran oil extract	120	2.87
Almond oil	**100**	**0.33**
Apricot kernel oil	**79**	**0.58**

Chemical group (color code)

Vitamin C	Sulfur compounds
Polyphenols	Dipeptide
Tannins	Carotenes
Terpenes	Seed oil

Antioxidant activity evaluation (EPR spectroscopy):

1. Antioxidant power (AP) — *in vitro*
2. Skin antioxidant protection (SAP) — *in vivo*
3. Radical Hair Protection Factor (RHF) — *in vivo*

The antioxidant unit (AU) is the antioxidant power of vitamin C solution at a concentration of 1 ppm:
AP (1 ppm vit C) = 1 AU

Figure III-1-6. Antioxidant power of various substances and mixtures

Protection of antioxidants against oxidation and degradation (secondary antioxidant protection)

Skincare products usually contain substances that can oxidize and lose their activity. These are primarily natural oils, especially those containing large amounts of different unsaturated fatty acids, as well as some fragrance components. Oxidized natural oils give off an unpleasant odor and become a source of peroxides and other toxic lipid peroxidation products, which can damage the skin and accelerate aging.

Butylated hydroxytoluene (BHT) and butylated hydroxyanisole (BHA) are most commonly used in cosmetic products because they have high antioxidant activity and are stable in most formulations. However, many consumers are suspicious of synthetic antioxidants and believe they can harm the skin. They are not even reassured by the fact that these substances are included in minute concentrations and that their level of safety is high.

In natural cosmetic formulations, vitamin E or its derivatives (e.g., tocopheryl acetate) and floretin (an antioxidant extracted from apple peel) protect easily oxidizable ingredients. A combination of three antioxidants — vitamin C, vitamin E, and ferulic acid — exhibits stability and good antioxidant activity.

Besides technical antioxidants that protect cosmetic ingredients from oxidation, the formulation includes compounds acting against prooxidants* and substances necessary for the body's own antioxidants:

- UV filters — reflect (zinc oxide, titanium dioxide) or absorb (e.g., methoxycinnamates, octocrylene, benzophenones) UV rays that provoke lipid peroxidation and other free-radical reactions
- Complexing agents (chelators) such as ethylenediaminetetraacetic acid (EDTA) — bind metal ions, including divalent iron ions, a strong prooxidant that triggers oxidative reactions in biosystems
- Cofactors of antioxidant enzymes — metal ions in the active centers of enzymes (selenium, copper, zinc, manganese)

---

* Pro-oxidants are chemicals that induce oxidative stress, either by generating reactive oxygen species or by inhibiting antioxidant systems. The oxidative stress produced by these chemicals can damage cells and tissues; for example, an overdose of the analgesic paracetamol (acetaminophen) can fatally damage the liver, partly through its ROS production.

1.4. Cosmetic camouflage

Foundation evens out the skin tone, which is particularly useful for those who are embarrassed about age spots. Modern foundations often contain moisturizers, anti-inflammatory agents, and UV filters, which increase their beneficial effect on skin prone to pigmentation. However, outdoors in sunny weather, this may not be enough to protect against UV light, so sunscreen is still applied on top of the foundation. Nowadays, there are UV sprays that don't require rubbing and can be used in such cases.

White spots in vitiligo can also be camouflaged with a traditional foundation, as well as using dihydroxyacetone (DHA) self-tanning products. DHA is a sugar that binds to amino acids in the *stratum corneum* to form colored conjugates that mimic a tan. The effect is visible a few hours after application. The product is applied several times a week until the desired effect is achieved since the pigmentation caused by DHA is reduced during physiological exfoliation of the *stratum corneum*. This method is not suitable for everyone and should only be used by individuals whose natural skin tone is close to that formed by DHA (European Guidelines for the Treatment of Dermatological Diseases, 2008).

More information about cosmetic ingredients and treatments is available in the *Comprehensive Cosmetic Skincare in Cosmetic Dermatology & Skincare Practice* and *Chemical Peeling in Cosmetic Dermatology & Skincare Practice* books.

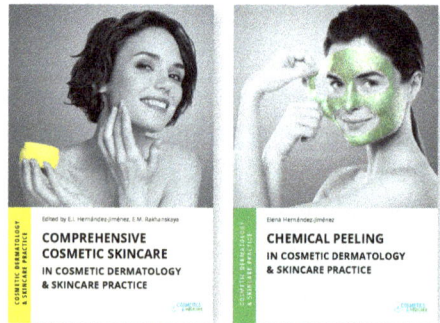

Edited by E.I. Hernández Jiménez, S.M. Rakhunskaya

COMPREHENSIVE COSMETIC SKINCARE
IN COSMETIC DERMATOLOGY & SKINCARE PRACTICE

Elena Hernández Jiménez

CHEMICAL PEELING
IN COSMETIC DERMATOLOGY & SKINCARE PRACTICE

Chapter 2
Energy-based technologies for treating pigmentation disorders

Along with the use of cosmetic products to eliminate pigment abnormalities, physical methods play a prominent role. The main "players" for treating pigment lesions — both superficial and deep — are lasers and intense pulsed light (IPL) devices, which can destroy the pigment and the cells containing it.

The other methods can be regarded as secondary — they cannot solve the problem of pigmented spots, but in general, they help to lighten the skin. These methods primarily include microdermabrasion, which removes the *stratum corneum*'s upper layers and stimulates the cell renewal in the epidermis. More traumatic dermabrasion affecting the living epidermis layers is rarely performed today because of the high risk of post-inflammatory dyschromia. In this regard, there are questions about the advisability of using radiofrequency (RF) technologies. Their effect is associated with thermal and, in the case of RF microneedling, mechanical damage and subsequent inflammation. Unlike selective pigment lasers, all skin cells are affected, not only those containing melanin. In some cases, low-intensity laser therapy (LLLT) is used as an auxiliary method. Below we consider it in a little more detail.

2.1. Light therapy

2.1.1. Skin preparation for laser treatment

Before talking about the features of light-based technologies in pigmentation treatment, **we emphasize the importance of skin pre- and post-treatment with topical agents**.

It is necessary to reduce the background activity of melanocytes, which is increased in the more pigmented areas. For this purpose, **antioxidant and anti-inflammatory agents, as well as sunscreens, must be used a few weeks before** the physical therapy, regardless of whether you use depigmenting agents or not. The energy-based methods are included in the treatment only after the first stage of therapy is successfully completed and the skin is ready for more intensive treatment. This may include LLLT session(s) to prevent inflammation.

Depigmenting topical agents can be continued/discontinued during the course, but **sun protection measures should always be taken**.

2.1.2. Mechanism of action

Attempts to use lasers to remove pigmented lesions were made almost immediately after their invention. In 1964, the founder of laser medicine, Leon Goldman, first used the ruby laser to remove nevi (Goldman L. et al., 1964). However, at that time, certain technical problems led to a high risk of scarring and dyschromia.

The situation improved dramatically after American scientists Richard Anderson and John Parrish developed the concept of **selective photothermolysis**. It is based on the fact that the structures contained in the skin absorb light of different wavelengths in different ways. By selecting light with a particular wavelength, it is possible to selectively affect specific targets containing many photosensitive substances — chromophores, which absorb certain light waves more intensely than their surroundings.

When a chromophore absorbs light energy, it goes into an excited state. This state is unstable, so the molecules quickly return to their usual form and emit excess energy in the form of heat. This results in the heating and destruction of both the chromophore itself and the cell (depending on the amount of transmitted energy) in which it is contained. Thus, it is possible to act only on structures with many chromophores while neighboring cells containing little or no chromophores remain unaffected.

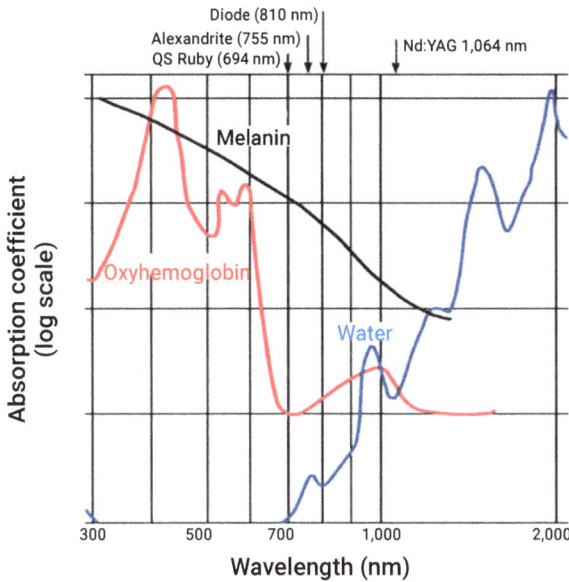

Figure III-2-1. Dependence of the absorption coefficient on the wavelength of laser radiation for different chromophores

Melanin is a chromophore. It actively absorbs light waves in the so-called "melanin window" range from 600 to 1100 nm (**Fig. III-2-1**). In this range, radiation is more actively "captured" by melanin, while the absorption coefficient (the intensity with which structures absorb light energy) of other chromophores, such as hemoglobin and water, is significantly lower. This makes it possible to target the pigmented formations directly, minimally affecting the surrounding structures.

The intensity of light energy absorption by melanin decreases as the radiation wavelength increases, but longer wavelengths allow deeper penetration into the skin. At the same time, shorter wavelengths can damage the surface pigment with relatively low energy, while longer wavelengths, although penetrating deeper, require more energy to cause damage to melanosomes. However, it is impossible to achieve an isolated effect on melanin by wavelength selection alone (optical selectivity). Although water and hemoglobin absorb radiation in the melanin window range less intensely than melanin, they still absorb it, especially if the defect is deep.

Therefore, another challenge arises — delivering the maximal number of photons to the target chromophore before they are "grabbed" by competing chromophores close to the target. This is possible by optimal selection of the pulse duration, which is determined by considering the **thermal relaxation time (TRT)**, the period required for the heated target to give up 63% of its heat to its surroundings. The pulse duration must be equal to, and ideally several times less than, the TRT of the target structure. Otherwise, it does not have time to cool down, and significant heat spreads to the adjacent non-target tissues, causing their thermal damage.

Since melanin and melanosomes containing melanin are very small, their destruction requires a short exposure. According to different data sources, the TRT of melanosomes ranges from 50 to 250 ns, so for their destruction to be effective and safe, the laser pulse duration must be in the nanosecond and even picosecond range. At the same time, the pulse energy must be high enough to destroy the target without overheating the surrounding structures.

2.1.3. Light technologies for treating pigmentary lesions

Today, the main lasers used for pigmented lesions are Q-switched (QS) lasers — nano- and picosecond lasers. This technology facilitates the generation of very short pulses with very high power. In skincare practice, these lasers are actively replacing long-pulsed lasers, as well as continuous-beam ablative lasers, because these types of exposure are associated with the risks of scarring and post-inflammatory hyperpigmentation. Destruction of melanin under the influence of ultrashort pulsed lasers is not only due to photothermolysis but also to the photoacoustic effect: rapid heating of tissues leads to shockwaves that "break" the pigment granules into fragments, which are then utilized by macrophages. The shorter the pulse duration, the more pronounced the photomechanical effect and the lower the photothermal effect.

Fractional ablative and non-ablative lasers (including a separate line to enhance penetration of depigmenting agents from the area of work), as well as IPL sources with filters to target the pigmented pathology, are also used to remove pigmented lesions (**Table III-2-1**).

Table III-2-1. Laser devices for the treatment of pigmentation disorders treatment

SELECTIVE SHORT-PULSED LASERS (NANO- AND PICOSECOND LASERS)	SELECTIVE LONG-PULSED LASERS AND IPL	FRACTIONAL LASERS	LASER RE-SURFACING WITH A SOLID LASER BEAM
• Copper vapor laser (511 nm)	• KTP (532 nm) • PDL (585–595 nm) • Alexandrite (755 nm) • IPL (560–1200 nm)	**Non-ablative fractionated lasers** (1540–1550 nm) **Ablative fractional lasers:** • Er:YSGG (2770 nm) • Er:YAG (2940 nm) • CO_2 (10,600 nm)	• Er:YSGG (2770 nm) • Er:YAG (2940 nm) • CO_2 (10,600 nm)
• QS KTP (532 nm) • QS Ruby (694 nm)			
• QS Alex (755/785 nm)			
• QS Nd:YAG (1064 nm)			
• Fractional nozzles for picosecond lasers (532/755/1064 nm)			

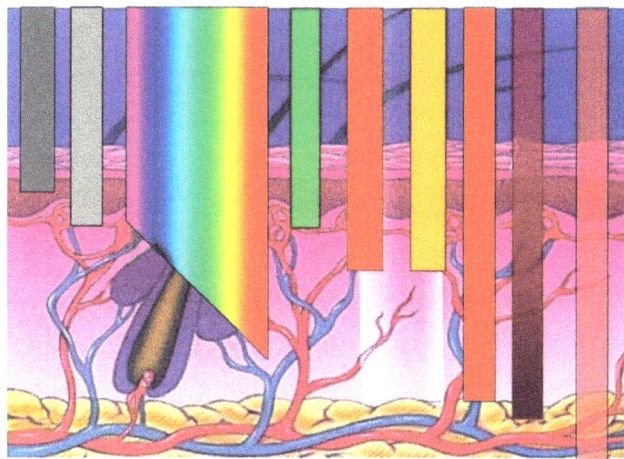

Figure III-2-2. Depth of penetration of different laser types depending on the wavelength

The choice of laser is determined primarily by the depth of the pigment (**Fig. III-2-2**) (see Part II, section 1.2).

Superficial epidermal lesions — laser radiation that has a high melanin absorption coefficient and low risk of competitive interaction can be used to remove them. These can be both long-pulsed and short-pulsed lasers, as well as IPL systems:

- Long-pulsed lasers — 511, 532, 585/595, 694, 755 nm
- QS lasers — 532, 755, 785, 1064 nm
- IPL — 560–1200 nm

Superficial epidermal lesions with keratosis (seborrheic or actinic keratosis) — require the destruction of not only pigment but also excess tissue, so the main method of their removal is ablative photothermolysis with a continuous or fractionated beam of erbium-doped yttrium aluminium garnet (Er:YAG) and CO_2 lasers.

Dermal pigmented defects require high-energy short-pulsed QS nanosecond and picosecond lasers operating at 755 and 1064 nm wavelengths. Resurfacing is contraindicated in the case of dermal defects.

Let's take a closer look at all these devices.

Green light

What does it work on? Green light's penetrating ability is relatively low, so its effect is limited to the epidermis. Therefore, lasers emitting in the green part of the spectrum may only be used to treat superficial epidermal hyperpigmentations (epidermal melasma, lentigos, freckles, café-au-lait spots, and Becker's nevi).

Devices: nanosecond copper vapor laser (511 nm), long-pulsed, and QS Nd:YAG/KTP (potassium titanyl phosphate) laser with doubled frequency (532 nm).

- **Copper vapor laser (511 nm).** Short nanosecond pulses of the copper vapor laser make it possible to produce both photoacoustic and photothermal destruction. The first mechanism mainly destroys melanin, while the second one destroys melanocytes. By varying the power and duration of pigment defect exposure, it is possible to adjust the ratios between these mechanisms. However, radiation at 511 nm cannot penetrate deep skin layers, so this laser can remove only superficial defects.
- **Long-pulsed and QS Nd:YAG laser with frequency-doubling capabilities (532 nm), so-called KTP laser.** Its radiation is absorbed by both melanin and hemoglobin and acts on the skin's

surface layers. Exposure to the QS KTP laser leads to melanosome destruction and more pronounced damage of melanocytes in general, in place of which the formation of new cells producing a normal amount of pigment is registered. It is recommended to use a low energy density. However, some studies have shown that long-pulsed KTP lasers are more effective in removing superficial pigmentations than short-pulsed QS laser devices.

Peculiarities of exposure. Using these lasers is undesirable in people with dark skin phototypes, as the radiation in the green part of the spectrum is extremely actively absorbed by melanin — burns, and additional changes in pigmentation (both hypo- and hyper-) are possible. Even in the case of an initial successful result, pigmentation defects may recur at a later date.

Since photons in this energy range are also well absorbed by hemoglobin, purpura, and small bruises may appear after using these lasers. Usually, they disappear 1–2 weeks after the procedure, but in some cases, post-inflammatory hyperpigmentation may develop in the place of bruises. Therefore, before treating large skin surfaces, experts recommend performing test procedures on small areas.

Yellow light

What does it work on? The penetration capacity of yellow light is higher than that of green light but is still low. Therefore, these lasers are also primarily used to correct epidermal defects.

Devices: long-pulsed dye laser (585–595 nm), PDL.

Exposure features. The wavelength of 585–595 nm is well absorbed mainly by hemoglobin, which is why PDL is the "gold standard" for treating vascular lesions. At these wavelengths, the radiation is also absorbed by melanin and is sometimes used to correct superficial pigmented defects. However, PDL is of particular interest for melasma, as increased vascularization is thought to play an important role in the pathogenesis of this disease. Receptors for the vascular growth factors VEGF-1 and VEGF-2, which can affect cell activity, have been found on the surface of melanocytes, so targeting the vascular component can reduce the stimulation of melanocyte activity and reduce pigmentation.

Red light

What does it work on? The red wavelengths penetrate deeper than those in the green part of the spectrum, allowing them to be used to correct both epidermal and dermal pigmented lesions.

Devices: QS ruby (694 nm) and QS alexandrite (755 nm) lasers.

- **QS Ruby laser (694 nm).** The ruby laser is used to treat a wide range of hyperpigmentation disorders (e.g., melasma, melanocytic nevi, lentigo, café-au-lait spots, nevi of Ota, chloasma, Becker's nevi). At the same time, the procedures are accompanied by a relatively low risk of adverse side effects (most of them are observed when using ruby laser for treating nevi of Ota). It can be assumed that the latter is related to higher energy levels used for dermal pigmentation treatment. This is also confirmed by the fact that even when the more gentle fractional QS ruby laser is used to treat superficial pigmentations in light skin phototypes, high energy densities lead to a significant increase in adverse events. Specialists suggest careful patient selection and more gentle procedures.

- **QS Alex laser (755 nm).** The the energy produced by Alex laser is less intensely absorbed by melanin than that obtained from the Ruby laser, so it can be used in patients with darker skin. However, experts recommend adhering to the principle of relatively low exposure dose and a limited number of treatments. QS nanosecond and picosecond alexandrite laser can remove lentigines, benign melanocytes, café-au-lait spots, nevi of Ota, and melasma.

Exposure features. In contrast to devices generating green light, these lasers do not cause bruising since red-band radiation is much less absorbed by hemoglobin. However, although the damage to melanocytes is substantial, relapses are also possible.

Near-IR light

What does it work on? The absorption intensity of near-infrared radiation by melanin is relatively low (less than for green and red spectral ranges). However, other chromophores, such as hemoglobin and water, absorb it even less intensely. This accounts for the high penetrating power of this radiation and the possibility of using it to treat deep dermal pigmentary defects.

Devices: QS Nd:YAG laser (1064 nm).

Exposure features. Ultra-short pulsed (nano- and picosecond) radiation with a wavelength of 1064 nm causes fragmentation and disintegration of melanin granules, sublethal damage of melanosomes, and release of pigment into the cell cytoplasm. Low melanin absorption coefficient allows the use of a low-dose QS Nd:YAG 1064 nm laser in people with dark skin phototypes — laser energy of this wavelength is poorly absorbed by epidermal pigment, thus reducing the risk of hypopigmentation and burns. Although 1064 nm radiation is generally less intense on pigmentary defects, the QS Nd:YAG laser is the primary choice in people with III−V skin phototypes.

Another feature of the QS Nd:YAG laser 1064 nm is its complex action — despite its radiation being most actively absorbed by melanin, it also acts on hemoglobin and water molecules. Therefore, along with the pigment destruction, there can be blood vessel coagulation (which is relevant, for example, in the case of excessive vascularization in melasma) and damage to collagen, resulting in dermal remodeling, rejuvenation, and improvement in the skin tone. The combination of these effects is used in the so-called "laser toning" procedure, popular in Asian countries.

In general, relatively long intervals between treatments and a limited number of procedures are recommended for treating pigmented lesions. Thus, the following parameters are often used for melasma patients: energy density — 2−4 J/cm^2, pulse duration — 5−12 ms, spot size — 6 mm, 5−10 sessions with an interval of one week.

Intense pulsed light (IPL)

What does it work on? The range of radiation generated by IPL devices (500−1200 nm) is absorbed by all the main chromophores of the skin — melanin, hemoglobin, and water. For a more targeted effect, special light filters are used. For example, 500−550 nm filters can be used to correct epidermal pigment defects, and long-wave filters can be used to target deeper accumulations of melanin.

Exposure features. Energy emitted by IPL devices is distributed among different chromophores, so it is relatively low for each individual type. Elevated light intensity is necessary to affect specific structures. However, it is fraught with undesirable side effects — the higher IPL energy densities allow more intensive effects and deeper treatment. Still, they are associated with the risk of burns and post-inflammatory hyperpigmentation in patients with darker skin phototypes. Therefore, the indications for IPL exposure are primarily superficial epidermal pigmented disorders. It should be noted that such procedures are often less effective than when using lasers operating in the green and red parts of the spectrum. At the same time, modern devices "bring" IPL technology closer to laser in its effectiveness in removing pigmented and vascular defects.

Laser resurfacing and fractional photothermolysis

What does it work on? The main target for laser resurfacing and fractional photothermolysis procedures is water, and since it is present in all cells and skin structures, not only melanocytes but all tissues are damaged. Accordingly, laser resurfacing is used less and less frequently to remove pigmented lesions and is advised only in the presence of hyperkeratotic lesions. However, even in this case, fractional lasers — which form many microthermal zones (MTZ) in the skin, surrounded by intact tissues — are preferable. The depth of their effect is adjustable: fractional lasers can be used for superficial and deep pigmentary lesions, particularly for lentigo, melasma, Becker's nevus, nevus of Ota, seborrheic keratosis, and post-inflammatory hyperpigmentation.

Devices and exposure features

For ablative fractional photothermolysis:

- CO_2 laser (10,600 nm)
- Er:YAG laser (2940 nm)

In ablative fractional photothermolysis, due to the high absorption coefficient of 2940 nm and 10,600 nm radiation by water, it evaporates almost immediately, even from those cells with low water content (such as those in the *stratum corneum*). Although the fractionated procedure is less traumatic than laser resurfacing, its implementation is also associated with the risk of post-inflammatory hyperpigmentation. Some experts recommend using this method only to remove small pigmented lesions such as lentigines, seborrheic keratoses, or hyperpigmentations resistant to other therapy types.

For non-ablative fractional photothermolysis (the *stratum corneum* remains intact):

- **Diode laser (1440 nm)** shows good results in the complex treatment of melasma:
  - three low-intensity treatments at three-week intervals
  - whitening creams (ascorbic and kojic acid-based in the morning and hydroquinone and 0.025% tretinoin-based in the evening)
  - weekly peels with 20% salicylic acid
- **Fractionated Nd:YAG laser (1440 nm)** has shown good results in the treatment of nevi of Ota that were resistant to previous treatments with the Nd:YAG laser (1064 nm).
- **Erbium laser (1550 nm)** — the following exposure parameters are used for melasma treatment: MTZ density — 2000–2500 per cm^2, 6–10 mJ per microbeam. Course of treatment: 3–4 treatments at intervals of 1–2 months. Good results (35–50% improvement on average) along with rare undesirable side effects are observed.
- **Thulium laser (1927 nm)** is characterized by the highest absorption by water molecules of all non-ablative lasers, so it is more effective in damaging epidermal pigments.

Non-ablative fractional photothermolysis relies on radiation in the 1300–2000 nm spectral range. Light waves in this spectrum have a lower absorption coefficient than the radiation of ablative lasers and heat the epidermis and dermis structures to 45–90 °C (coagulation). It is recommended for the treatment of dermal and mixed-pigmented lesions, heterogeneous skin tone, and melasma.

Since melasma formation (and according to some data, post-inflammatory hyperpigmentation as well) has vascular causes, some specialists recommend combining non-ablative fractional photothermolysis with selective PDL (510 nm) or Nd:YAG laser with double frequency (532 nm) for better results.

2.1.4. Low-level laser radiation

In addition to high-level lasers, low-level laser therapy (LLLT) — with much lower energy and power of laser light than in the devices discussed above — is also used in skincare practice. Such low-intensity laser radiation in the red or near-infrared range (630–1000 nm) is used to modulate (stimulate or inhibit) the functional activity of cells — to achieve a positive therapeutic effect. Procedures performed using LLLT are known as **photobiomodulation** (aka **photomodulation**).

Although the mechanisms of LLLT action are still not precisely defined, the mitochondrial theory is considered the most valid. According to this theory, red and near-IR LLLT radiation is absorbed by the key enzyme of the mitochondrial respiratory chain — the cytochrome C oxidase enzyme. This triggers a cascade of events leading to the biostimulation of various processes.

Numerous studies have demonstrated anti-inflammatory, wound healing, stimulating, immunomodulating, and lipolytic effects of LLLT. Accordingly, in skincare practice, this type of exposure is used to treat inflammatory diseases (e.g., acne, atopic dermatitis, eczema, psoriasis), to accelerate healing after aggressive procedures and normalize scar healing, as well as stimulate the renewal of epidermal and dermal structures, for lipolysis, and in alopecia treatment.

As for treating pigmentary disorders, low-intensity laser therapy is used mainly as an adjunctive method — to reduce inflammation. In this respect, LLLT can be considered as prevention of post-inflammatory pigmentation, especially in combination with topical antioxidants. Moreover, some researchers claim that LLLT can have a direct inhibitory effect on melanogenesis, even though LLLT of practically the same wavelength is used for vitiligo repigmentation. In addition, as we said above, IR radiation can stimulate ROS formation, which hypothetically could contribute to the stimulation of melanogenesis.

Thus, it is worth repeating that the fundamental molecular and cellular mechanisms responsible for the LLLT effects have not yet been definitively determined. In addition, LLLT exhibits a dual effect, which is why the procedures involving this device are called photobiomodulation rather than photostimulation or photoinhibition. There are unambiguous differences in the effects of low-intensity laser exposure depending on the wavelength used and the small variations in radiation doses. As a result, the desired stimulation can turn into undesirable inhibition and vice versa. We can get no effect at all or have a damaging impact. But even if these doses are evaluated as a part of academic research (studies on anti-inflammatory procedures are currently only being conducted in the context of melanogenesis regulation), it is far from certain that they can be achieved in reality. In sum, good effects can only be attained with certified devices, using appropriate radiation parameters while adhering to the protocols of the procedures precisely.

2.1.5. Effectiveness of laser treatment in pigmentation disorders

The experience of a large number of specialists shows that different pigmented lesions respond differently to high-intensity laser treatment — summarized in **Table III-2-2** and **III-2-3**.

When using lasers to remove melanocytic nevi, it is essential to be sure that they are indeed benign. There is no evidence to suggest that laser exposure can induce malignant cell rearrangement. Still, there is a large body of data on the removal of existing undiagnosed skin cancer with benign protocols, followed by more active growth or late diagnosis problems.

Table III-2-2. The expected response of pigmented desorders to laser treatment

GOOD RESPONSE	MODERATE RESPONSE	VARIABLE RESPONSE	CONFLICTING RESULTS
• Lentigo • Freckles • Seborrheic keratoses • Nevus of Ota • Nevus of Ito	• Melasma • Post-inflammatory hyper-pigmentation	• Café-au-lait spots • Spotted nevus • Becker's nevus	Congenital and acquired melanocytic nevi (risk of incomplete destruction and removal of deep nevus cells)

Table III-2-3. Estimated efficacy of phototherapy depending on the pigment localization

DEVICE	PIGMENT LOCALIZATION		
	EPIDERMAL	MIXED	DERMAL
QS Copper vapor laser (511 nm)	+++	++	+
Long-pulsed and QS Nd:YAG laser with doubled frequency (532 nm)/KTP	+++	++	+
QS Ruby laser (694 nm)	+++	+++	++
QS Alex laser (755 nm)	++	+++	++
QS Nd:YAG laser (1064 nm)	+	+++	+++
IPL	+++	+++	+
Ablative fractional photothermolysis	+++	+	+
Non-ablative fractional photothermolysis	+	++	+++

Therefore, in the case of removing pigmented lesions, primary diagnosis and dermatoscopy, in addition to clinical examination, are extremely important. In any suspicious cases, histological examination should be performed, and other methods of pigment defect removal should be chosen.

In cases where the decision to have a laser removal is made, it is recommended to excise the mass with a scalpel or scissors, send the tissue for histological analysis, and only when absence of malignancy is confirmed remove the remaining pigment with a laser. But there are also problems in this case — the excised tissue may not include a malignant nodus,, and the diagnosis will be erroneous. Therefore, where there are doubts, it is better not to proceed with the laser removal of a pigmented mass.

Understanding the capabilities of modern laser technology will help ensure a more correct device selection depending on the disorder type and increase the efficacy and safety of procedures.

Light technologies do not always provide safe and complete elimination of pigment spots. Still, they yield good results for practically all dyschromia types and are especially useful for deep pigment deposits where topical means are ineffective. Combining laser methods with topical agents — depigmenting and lightening — gives better results than monotherapy with any of the approaches. Moreover, combining adequate preparation and rehabilitation with an integrated approach also solves complex problems better.

Detailed information about light therapy is available in the *Lasers in Cosmetic Dermatology & Skincare Practice* book.

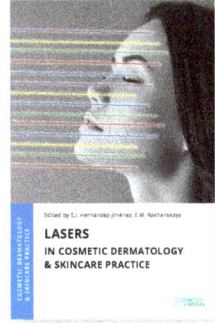

2.2. Mechanical methods

In the case of pigment defects, mechanical methods are used to remove surface corneocytes and accelerate the epidermis renewal, eliminating excessive pigment-loaded cells.

Another positive effect is that the removal of superficial layers improves the skin's permeability to topical preparations. Consequently, if depigmenting and lightening agents are used after the procedure, they will better penetrate the epidermis.

2.2.1. Microdermabrasion

The basis of dermabrasion is mechanical destruction of the skin with hard materials — layer-by-layer skin resurfacing with abrasive milling materials that separate the upper layers of the keratinized epithelium. The smaller the size of the abrasive particles, the less traumatic the procedure. Microdermabrasion is the gentlest option for the treatment of pigmented blemishes.

Microdermabrasion (or mechanical peeling) is a gentle and painless way to remove dead skin cells and stimulate skin regeneration. It is used not only to treat pigmentation but is also very effective as an element of a comprehensive course aimed at removing scars of different origin, tattoos, acne, warts, spider veins, deep wrinkles, including those in the nasolabial triangle, and other defects.

In addition to accelerating exfoliation, temporary removal of the *stratum corneum* opens an opportunity for skincare specialists to deliver the necessary substances with a specific action to the deep skin layers. As shown in experiments on hairless rats (Zhou Y., Banga A.K., 2011), penetration of hydrophilic substances increases immediately after the first microdermabrasion procedure and linearly increases with the number of passages. Recovery of the initial level of permeability for the hydrophilic dye calcein occurs about 96 h after microdermabrasion. So, the first three days after the procedure provide an opportunity for facilitated delivery of hydrophilic substances into the dermis.

Another modern type of dermabrasion is **sandblasting microdermabrasion**, which is performed by treating the skin surface with a jet of microcrystalline powder (typically using aluminum oxide). However, some devices use microcrystals of sodium bicarbonate (soda), sodium chloride (table salt), and magnesium oxide (burnt magnesia). Mechanical removal of skin scales opens pores of sebaceous and sweat glands and helps to renew the cell composition of the epidermis. The pressure of the particle jet on the skin reflexively stimulates microcirculation in the deep layers of the skin. All this improves the skin condition by smoothing the unevenness of its relief, removing keratinized masses, and increasing turgor.

Another type of microdermabrasion, the so-called **diamond resurfacing**, is performed using rotating nozzles with diamond coating and vacuum suction, which are used to remove the surface keratinized skin layers gently. It is a superficial procedure and can be performed on the face, neck, décolletage, and other parts of the body, as well as any skin type.

2.2.2. Gas–liquid microdermabrasion

This technology combines three methods of exposure:
1. Mechanical crystal-free exfoliation
2. Moderate vacuum
3. Multifunctional skincare serums

Its destructive component (mechanical exfoliation) is not very pronounced but is still of key importance. Exfoliation occurs thanks to special nozzles with different surface shapes: rapid movements of the applicator with the appropriate nozzle across the skin delicately "scrape" corneocytes and surface impurities.

The applicator design allows a solution to flow into the nozzle during exfoliation, delivering it to the skin through special holes. Serum flow is only possible when the nozzle is in contact with the skin — when there is no contact, the serum is not discharged and, therefore, is not wasted.

Vacuum (besides the technical function of controlling the serum flow) has a pronounced trophic-stimulating effect on the skin: capillary depots are opened, metabolic processes in the skin are activated, lymphatic drainage improves skin tone, and muscles that are woven into the dermis increase in volume, resulting in a lifting effect. Besides, the vacuum perfectly cleanses pores. When working with such pigmented defects as post-acne spots, the vacuum has a resolving and de-fibrosing impact, i.e., it prevents the formation of pronounced fibrotic changes and improves blood circulation, which eliminates the vascular component of the spot.

Chapter 3
Injectable methods

Some pigmentation treatment protocols include injectable methods such as microneedling, mesotherapy, biorevitalization, and platelet-rich plasma (PRP) therapy. We want to emphasize that all injectable methods are associated with skin damage. As noted earlier, any skin damage is a risk factor for developing post-inflammatory hyperpigmentation. While in the case of lasers and IPL devices, we use aggressive action to directly destroy melanin and melanocytes, and such aggression is justified even though it is associated with risks, injectable methods alone do not produce depigmentation. However, they can provide some additional benefits in treating pigmentation. Still, before deciding on this mode of treatment, one must weigh the risks and benefits very carefully. Let's discuss these methods.

1.1. Microneedling

Mesotherapy is a method of treatment that involves the delivery of active substances into the deeper skin layers via intradermal or subcutaneous injection. A syringe, mesoinjector, mesoroller (dermaroller), or dermapen is used for this purpose (**Fig. III-3-1**).

When using mesoroller or dermapen treatment, multiple punctures are formed in the skin through which substances pre-applied to its surface pass (that is why the procedure using the dermaroller is also called microneedle therapy or microneedling). It is also possible to apply active ingredients after the procedure — the skin permeability in the puncture point remains elevated for some time. **Microneedling is the most common injectable method of pigmentation treatment; the other options are used much less frequently.**

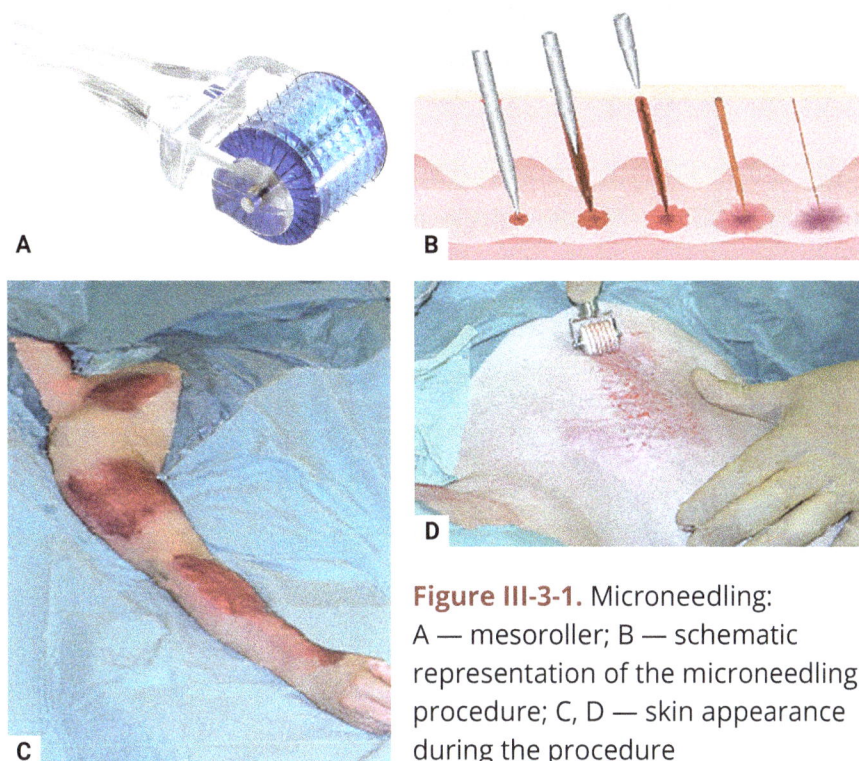

Figure III-3-1. Microneedling: A — mesoroller; B — schematic representation of the microneedling procedure; C, D — skin appearance during the procedure

In the case of pigmentary disorders, microneedling is used to deliver substances with depigmenting and brightening effects — tranexamic acid, vitamin C; previously, hydroquinone and peeling agents into deep skin layers (Budamakuntla L. et al., 2013; Hou A. et al., 2017; Ismail E.S.A. et al., 2019; Menon A. et al., 2019). Such delivery can be justified in the case of deep pigmentary lesions when melanin is found in the dermal layer of the skin, where most topical agents cannot penetrate on their own.

Typically, microneedling is used for mixed or deep melasma in people with dark skin phototypes (Ramaut L. et al., 2018). Microneedling with lightening agents is also sometimes used for people with light phototypes and superficial forms of pigmentation (Ismail E.S.A. et al., 2019). However, given the additional trauma to the basal membrane and the dermal layer, this approach may not be justified in the absence of problems in the deep layers. As vitamin C can penetrate the living layers of the epidermis on its own, it is debatable if creating an additional stress load on melanocytes is beneficial in these individuals.

Given the availability of lasers and IPL devices in the arsenal of modern cosmetic dermatology, which allows one to "get" the pigment at any level of occurrence, microneedling should be considered an economically cheaper way to affect the deep pigment when laser use is not possible. At the same time, it is much less targeted while increasing the risk of post-inflammatory hyperpigmentation.

1.2. Biorevitalization

Biorevitalization is a method of intradermal injection of native high-molecular-weight hyaluronic acid to restore the physiological environment and normalize metabolic processes in the dermal layer.

Although biorevitalization procedures lighten the skin (Sparavigna A. et al., 2015), the exact mechanisms behind this effect are yet to be fully elucidated. It is known that the effect of hyaluronic acid (HA) depends on its molecular weight. For instance, high-molecular-weight native HA (mass over 500 kDa) has antioxidant, anti-inflammatory, and immunomodulatory properties and controls many biological and biochemical processes, including inflammation and immune responses. It can thus be assumed that the normalization of metabolic processes in the dermal layer helps reduce the transmission of stress signals to melanocytes, including reducing the effects of psychological stress on the skin.

It is also known that medium-molecular-weight HA can stimulate the proliferation of fibroblasts and keratinocytes by binding to CD44 receptors on the cell surface, which may help accelerate epidermal renewal and exfoliation of pigment-laden corneocytes (Kaya G. et al., 2006).

In addition, optical brightening can be observed by moisturizing the skin and smoothing out surface wrinkles. Moistened skin simply reflects light better.

However, skin brightening after biorevitalization treatment is more of a secondary, although pleasant, addition to the rejuvenation effect and maintenance of skin health rather than an indication to use the method for the treatment of pigmentation.

1.3. PRP (platelet-rich plasma) therapy

PRP therapy is a modern method of treatment based on the use of autologous platelet-rich plasma obtained from the patient's whole blood.

PRP contains more than 30 bioactive substances: growth factors, adhesive molecules, and cytokines that stimulate tissue-healing reactions, metabolic and anabolic processes, and have an anti-inflammatory effect. The main ones are platelet-derived growth factor (PDGF), epidermal growth factor (EGF), fibroblast growth factor (FGF), vascular endothelial growth factor (VEGF), hepatocyte growth factor (HGF), transforming growth factor (TGFβ), serotonin, histamine, dopamine, and ATP.

Besides the ability to reduce inflammation and activate metabolic processes, which can reduce the stress load on fibroblasts, as in the case of biorevitalization, some of the mentioned growth factors directly affect melanogenesis processes. However, they can both inhibit and activate melanin formation. Therefore, there is evidence in the literature both about the brightening effects of PRP (Cayırlı M. et al., 2014; Sirithanabadeekul P. et al., 2020) and its ability to exacerbate pigmentation (Uysal C.A., Ertas N.M., 2017).

Injectable methods can indeed be adjunctive for pigmentation treatment and skin lightening but are not the methods of choice. Their use is recommended before laser or phototherapy to increase the skin's regenerative potential. They must be used **carefully** since trauma from multiple punctures inevitably causes inflammation, which can activate melanocytes.

Chapter 4
Nutraceuticals for skin lightening

Some of the active ingredients mentioned in the section on cosmetics (see Part III, chapter 1) can enhance the effects of topical whitening and brightening agents when taken systemically — such as oral medications and supplements. Some of the most popular compounds with proven effects in clinical trials include glutathione, *Polypodium leucocotmos* fern extract, and tranexamic acid (Mohiuddin A.K., 2019).

4.1. Glutathione

Glutathione is an antioxidant synthesized in our body from three amino acids: glutamine, cysteine, and glycine. It can also come from food (e.g., watermelon, avocado, broccoli, spinach, tomato).

Glutathione reduces skin pigmentation by disrupting cellular tyrosine transport. It also inactivates tyrosinase by binding copper ions required for this enzyme to work. Part of glutathione's brightening effect is also due to its antioxidant properties. The main problem with glutathione, when taken orally, is its hydrolysis by liver enzymes, resulting in the loss of its activity. Therefore, it has to be taken in high doses. Glutathione can also be injected.

The effectiveness of glutathione in brightening pigmentation has been confirmed in double-blind, placebo-controlled studies. In one such study, a noticeable effect occurred after four weeks of taking the drug at a dose of 500 mg/day (Arjinpathana N., Asawanonda P., 2012). The effectiveness of taking 250 mg of glutathione daily for 12 weeks has also been shown (Weschawalit S. et al., 2017).

The systemic use of the drug does not cause toxic effects (Al Ghamdi K.M. et al., 2020). However, high doses are still not advised — recent studies have demonstrated that oral administration of excessive amounts of antioxidants can contribute to the development and progression of cancer (Wiel C. et al., 2019).

Glutathione is usually combined with vitamin C, α-lipoic acid, and N-acetylcysteine (although there is no clinical confirmation of the effectiveness of N-acetylcysteine yet).

4.2. *Polypodium leucotomos* fern extract

Polypodium leucotomos fern extract is a strong antioxidant that inhibits oxidative stress and lipid peroxidation, reduces oxidative DNA damage by forming 8-hydroxy-2-deoxyguanosine, and inhibits pyrimidine dimer accumulation. In addition, it decreases the levels of proinflammatory cytokines and transcription factors, cyclooxygenase 2 and nitric oxide synthase, protects Langerhans cells, inhibits glutathione oxidation in cells, and inhibits trans-urocanic acid photoisomerization (Nestor M. et al., 2014).

The systemic effects of *P. leucotomos* extract have long been studied. Since the effects of natural extracts can vary greatly depending on the extraction method and the concentration of active agents, it should be noted that Fernblock® (standardized aqueous extract of the *P. leucotomos* fern; IFC/Cantabria Labs, Spain) was examined in most published studies (Del Rosso J.Q., 2019). When taken orally, the extract provides a sun-protective effect: it reduces IPD reactions, increases the minimal erythema dose, and reduces sensitivity to the sun (Nestor M. et al., 2014). It is also used to reduce the phototoxic effects of PUVA therapy and prevent photodermatosis (Middelkamp-Hup M.A. et al., 2004; Choudhry S.Z. et al., 2014). In addition, double-blind placebo-controlled studies have shown its ability to reduce the severity of melasma (Goh C.-L. et al., 2018). It is suggested that due to its pronounced anti-inflammatory effect, oral forms of *P. leucotomos* extract can also be used to prevent post-inflammatory hyperpigmentation (Juhasz M.L.W., Levin M.K., 2018; Krutmann J. et al., 2020).

4.3. Tranexamic acid

Skin lightening using tranexamic acid systemically was the starting point for the study of its bleaching properties (which we described in detail in the section on depigmenting agents, see Part III, section 1.1).

However, since tranexamic acid also has other systemic effects, such as antifibrinolytic, its oral forms are only used as an additional method in treating complex pigmentary lesions, particularly resistant forms of melasma, and only if there are no contraindications.

In the case of melasma, tranexamic acid not only exhibits depigmenting and anti-inflammatory effects but also exerts influence on the vascular component of the pathology. In particular, its ability to inhibit the synthesis of endothelial growth factors regulating angiogenesis and endothelin-1, which can directly affect melanocytes, is noteworthy (Kim S.J. et al., 2016). A systematic review of studies on oral forms of tranexamic acid confirmed its effectiveness even at low doses — taking a 250 mg daily dose produced noticeable effects after four weeks of therapy (Sarma N. et al., 2017). None of the studies reported significant adverse events, except for one case of deep vein thrombosis in a patient with existing protein S deficiency (Lee H.C. et al., 2016). Only mild gastrointestinal disturbances and changes in the menstrual cycle have been noted. Although extant research shows that tranexamic acid does not increase the risk of thromboembolism, the drug's prescription should be accompanied by a thorough pre-examination for contraindications and risk factors.

Some photoprotective and brightening effects of oral forms of carotenoids, niacinamide, ginseng, melatonin, and vitamins C and E have also been identified, but further research is required to corroborate these findings (Forbat E. et al., 2017; Juhasz M.L.W., Levin M.K., 2019; Krutmann J. et al., 2020).

Thus, some orally administered compounds with depigmenting, brightening, sun protection, and anti-inflammatory properties can provide additional benefits when their use is included in a comprehensive program for treating pigmentary lesions.

Part IV

Vitiligo

Hypomelanosis is a skin condition characterized by a focal decrease in melanin caused by genetic or specific physical (UV exposure) factors. One of the most common hypomelanoses is vitiligo. Vitiligo is a widespread pathology — it affects up to 1% of people in the world, and about 8% of the population of India. However, vitiligo is more common among young people — the average age of onset is about 29 years. Although it is not life-threatening, it has an extremely negative effect on the mental state of patients.

Vitiligo is an acquired disease, but the predisposition for this condition can be inherited. The pigment disappearance in specific areas of the skin is thought to occur due to certain drugs and chemicals, neurotrophic, neuroendocrine, and autoimmune factors of melanogenesis, as well as after inflammatory and necrotic processes in the skin.

The nature of vitiligo is not fully understood, and a reliable treatment method has not yet been found. Many believe vitiligo cannot be cured, but this is not true. Yes, it is difficult to treat, and it is not always possible to achieve complete repigmentation, but time is of the essence, and new therapeutic protocols are gradually emerging. Many of the currently used therapy modes involve the use of systemic drugs, tissue engineering, and surgical methods.

The challenges in treating vitiligo are as follows:
- Arresting the progression
- Achieving repigmentation
- Attaining a reduction in the recurrence rate
- Ensuring moral support for the sick
- Conducting educational work with patients and the community

In addition to practicing dermatologists, the Vitiligo Research Foundation supports patients with vitiligo and carries out educational work. Psychological support is essential, and in recent years there has been a noticeable destigmatization of the disease. Unfortunately, in some parts of the world this is still not the case.

Let us briefly describe the methods used in the treatment of vitiligo.

1.1. Light therapy

Phototherapy methods for vitiligo are classified as follows:
- Narrow-band UVB (311 nm) — general, local, and focused
- Excimer laser radiation
- UVA (PUVA therapy, general and local)
- Helium-neon (He-Ne) laser radiation
- CO_2 laser radiation (fractional exposure)
- Photodynamic therapy (PDT)
- Heliotherapy

1.1.1. Narrow-band UVB (311 nm)

Its effect is immunosuppression (stopping melanocyte destruction), stimulation of melanocyte growth factors (bFGF, endothelin), and stem cell activation. The effectiveness of narrow-band UVB radiation (UVB part of the spectrum) is also associated with the stimulation of follicular melanocytic stem cell migration into the epidermis, their differentiation, and proliferation, which is expressed in perifollicular repigmentation (Goldstein N.B. et al., 2015). The initial irradiation dose is 0.075 J/cm^2, increasing by 20% each session until mild erythema is achieved. Procedures are performed 2–3 times per week; the course lasts 6–12 months. Irradiation is combined with oral antioxidant intake.

1.1.2. Focused microphototherapy (Bioskin Evolution®)

This is targeted irradiation of depigmentation areas with narrow-band UVB laser energy by selectively directing light to white areas through an 1-cm diameter optical fiber emitter. It can be effective for segmental vitiligo. Irradiation is performed daily for 20–30 days.

1.1.3. B-band (XeCl) narrow-band UVB (308 nm) excimer laser

It is considered safer than narrow-band phototherapy, and its effective dose in segmental vitiligo is lower. An excimer lamp is also used as a light source, giving indirect and incoherent light with a wavelength of 308 nm — monochromatic 308 nm-excimer radiation. The disadvantages are the limited exposure area and the high cost of the procedures.

1.1.4. PUVA therapy

As its name suggests, PUVA therapy combines oral administration of a photosensitizer (psoralen) and UVA irradiation of the whole body, which is effective in 30–60% of cases. **Local PUVA therapy** (with external application of photosensitizer and irradiation of limited skin areas) is less effective. There is also **bath PUVA therapy** — the patient takes a bath with a photosensitizer dissolved in water before irradiation. The sun can be used instead of an artificial radiation source, but it is less effective than the traditional approach.

General PUVA therapy is used when more than 10% of the skin surface is affected. One type of combination of photosensitizer and UV radiation is called **KUVA therapy**. Here khellin, a plant substance from the Mediterranean plant *Ammi visnaga*, is used as a photosensitizer.

1.1.5. Photodynamic therapy

Photodynamic therapy (PDT) is a treatment method using photosensitizers and visible light of a specific wavelength. The photosensitizer is injected into the body intravenously, by application, or orally and then selectively accumulates in the target tissues (cells). As photosensitizers, 5-aminolevulinic acid (ALA) and methyl ester of ALA (MAL) are most commonly used; less frequently, though effectively, hypericin, chlorophyll, indocyanine green, and indolyl-3-acetic acid are used.

PDT is widely used to treat inflammatory skin diseases (psoriasis, acne, sarcoidosis), infectious pathologies (warts, *condyloma acuminata*, *cutaneous leishmaniasis*), and senile keratosis. PDT has been proven effective in treating precancerous conditions and superficial malignant skin tumors. PDT can also stimulate immune cells and inflammatory mediators with immunomodulatory effects, activating local–specific immunity. In addition, when used for PDT, radiation such as the low-energy helium-neon (He-Ne) laser (633 ± 10 nm) improves melanocyte adhesion to type IV collagens, inhibits their motility, and increases their migration on type I collagens and expression of α2β1 integrins, which promotes melanocyte proliferation (Lan C.C. et al., 2009).

Heliotherapy is used in countries with a lot of sunlight, where the population cannot afford physiotherapy procedures. For example, in Central Asia, parsley juice is used as a mild photosensitizer, vitamin E is given one hour before sun exposure, and radiation exposure is dosed, starting with 5 minutes and gradually increasing the duration to 15–30 minutes (in the presence of erythema, exposure duration is not increased). Salt baths reduce the UV load.

The undesirable effects of phototherapy are erythema, burns, telangiectasia, photoaging, hyperpigmentation of unaffected skin areas, phototoxicity, and carcinogenesis.

During treatment, some areas, predominantly the hands and feet, are less amenable to repigmentation. This may be due to the lower density of melanocytes, fewer stem cells, and lower levels of regulatory factors in these parts of the body (Esmat S.M. et al., 2012). We cannot ignore the fact that the maturation and function of stem cells are regulated not only by UV radiation but also by dermal fibroblasts, adipocytes, and hair follicle papilla cells.

1.1.6. Sunscreens

This new narrow-band phototherapy method occupies an intermediate place between photo- and pharmacotherapy. Its essence is as follows: the patient receives a cream that transmits only UV light with a wavelength of 311 nm, i.e., the person is actually "treated by the sun." Together with the cream, a program is sent to the patient's smartphone, determining how long the patient can stay in the sun for the optimal therapeutic effect.

1.2. Pharmacotherapy

Both systemic and topical agents are used in modern pharmaco-therapy, including:

- **Glucocorticosteroids** — topically and orally in the form of mini-pulse therapy
- **Neovir** — a systemic immunomodulator
- **Minocycline** — an antibiotic with anti-inflammatory, immu-nomodulatory, antioxidant, and anti-apoptotic properties. Re-cently, it has been considered an alternative means for arresting the vitiligo progression and stimulating repigmentation.
- **Vitamin D** (calcipotriol) — used in combination with external glucocorticosteroids, narrow-band UVB, and excimer laser and in high doses (35,000 IU per day) as monotherapy (Finamor D.C. et al., 2013).
- **Placenta extract** — here we mean Melagenin lotion plus, pref-erably in combination with narrow-band UVB 311 nm photother-apy. Due to the biological origin of the product, there is a risk of transmission of infections.
- **Afamelanotide (melanotan I)** — a synthetic analog of melano-cortin (α-melanocyte-stimulating hormone), a new concept in the treatment of vitiligo. Sold under the brand name Scenesse, this medication is used to prevent phototoxicity and to reduce pain from light exposure for people with erythropoietic proto-porphyria. It is an MC1R agonist and a synthetic peptide and ana-log of α-MSH. It is administered as subcutaneous implant.
- **Calcipotriol cream and ointment** — products containing vita-min D for topical application, can be used on their own or as a part of combination therapy.
- **Calcineurin inhibitors** — tacrolimus ointment (Protopik 0.1% and 0.03%) or pimecrolimus cream (Elidel) are used twice daily for 3–6 months. Both drugs are local immunomodulators and inhibit calcineurin action, preventing the activation of T-cells and their production of inflammatory cytokines.

Other systemic pharmacological methods include L-phenylalanine, *Polypodium leucotomos* and Gingko biloba fern extracts, vitamins B_{12},

C, and E, folic acid, and zinc as monotherapy or in combination with other treatments. Promising new drugs include Janus kinase inhibitors (JAK), interleukin inhibitors, and bimatoprost. There are active studies on their effectiveness and safety (Dina Y. et al., 2019).

1.3. Cosmetic and nutraceutical ingredients

There are cosmetic preparations and dietary supplements on the market that are recommended for vitiligo patients. Their composition includes antioxidants, vitamins, trace elements, and enzymes — an example is shown in **Table IV-1**.

Table IV-1. Some cosmetic preparations and dietary supplements used in the treatment of vitiligo

PRODUCT NAME	ACTIVE INGREDIENTS
Vitisking gel	Superoxide dismutase, copper, zinc, vitamin B_{12}
Vitasan	Extracts of St. John's wort, beggarticks, calendula, and walnut, fir oil, cedar oil
Vitix gel	Superoxide dismutase and catalase
Vitix tablets	Vitamins C, E, B_9, B_{12} and minerals Se, Cu, Zn
Vitices capsules	Borage oil, L-cysteine, vitamins E, B_{12}, melon extract, folic acid
Vitices gel	Lactoferrin, lactoperoxidase, calcium, superoxide dismutase, sea thistle, *Ginkgo biloba*, and Asian centella extracts
VitiLemna gel	*Lemna minor* extract
Baidianfeng Jiaonang capsules	Psoralea seeds, astragalus root, angelica etc.
Vitisteel tablets	Stellate amaranth extract, amaranth

Antioxidants (herbal extracts, vitamins) have an effect only in low doses, and vitamin E can reduce the impact of phototherapy altogether.

In folk medicine, various plants are used: rhubarb root juice, melon juice, a decoction of St. John's wort, garlic, and a small caddis.

Sirtuins (from Silent Information Regulator) — "longevity proteins" suppressing cellular apoptosis — have become a new trend in skincare and dermatology. Seven known sirtuins are expressed in the epidermis and derma, but SIRT1 is the most studied. The action of sirtuins relates to photoaging, inflammation, cancer development, and skin infections. These proteins are activated by resveratrol contained in grape peel and seeds, and red wine. Perhaps their use will be a new way to protect epidermal cells from damage (Becatti M. et al., 2014).

1.4. Surgical methods

Today, surgery is used in dermatological treatment only in cases where other methods have failed. However, regenerative medicine methods using cell technologies have great prospects. The main disadvantages are pain and the need for rehabilitation.

Currently, the main surgical methods used in the treatment of vitiligo are:

- Hair grafting
- Minipunch grafts
- Suction blister epidermal grafts (SBEG)
- Split-thickness skin grafts according to Tiersch
- Micrographs of hair follicles
- Cell suspension transplantation (keratinocytes, melanocytes, hair follicle cells)

In parallel, a new therapy concept is developing — **traumatizing vitiligo lesions** (dermabrasion, laser ablation, microneedling) to activate metabolic processes and cytokine production in response to trauma.

1.5. Depigmentation

Sometimes it is easier to depigment the remaining areas rather than return color to areas affected by vitiligo. This approach is used when the lesion is large in general or locally (e.g., the body has normal pigmentation, but 90% of the face is discolored). For lightening the stained areas, selective QS pigment lasers are currently recommended (see Part III, section 2.1).

1.6. Cosmetic camouflage

Cosmetic camouflage for hypopigmentation can be temporary or permanent (tattooing). When selecting temporary camouflage, there are difficulties with color matching, different textures of the applied products and the surrounding skin, resistance to sweat and water exposure, challenges with application and removal, and differences in tolerability. With tattooing, vitiligo must be in stable condition. In addition, even with a perfect color match, there may be a difference in tanning and repigmentation.

In general, tattooing is possible on small areas of the skin, and if the disease progresses and foci are unstable, it is better to use a temporary camouflage. The most well-known products developed for this purpose are Viticolor gel, Vitiligo Cover lotion, Dye-O-Derm, Dermask lotion, and Dermablend fluid.

1.7. Treatment efficacy and prognosis

Different lesions are known to respond differently to therapy. The treatment efficacy depends on the localization and area of the skin lesion. Complete repigmentation sometimes occurs spontaneously in limited lesions. Generalized vitiligo is rarely completely repigmented, and 15–30% of patients do not respond to therapy at all. Repigmentation of > 75% of the lesion area is considered a significant improvement.

It is rare enough to achieve complete repigmentation of the hands, and leukotrichia (graying of the hair) is considered a poor prognostic sign for any vitiligo area.

Thus, treating this pathology is possible, although it may require considerable effort. Of course, a dermatologist can perform pathogenetic treatments in individuals that do not respond to the skincare methods. Another option is laser treatment. Finally, skincare is advised after aggressive dermatological and surgical techniques, but psychological support for vitiligo patients is always essential.

Conclusion

The emergence of new data on the life of melanocytes makes it increasingly important to treat these cells with respect and caution, especially considering their neuroglial origin. Ill-informed and ill-considered interference with the process of natural skin pigmentation can lead to the most unfortunate consequences. This applies both to bleaching ethnic skin and to the pursuit of a bronze tan in people with white skin.

Melanocytes should be kept in mind not only when whitening with topical preparations but also with any cosmetic procedures that can be perceived by skin cells as external aggression. When skin cells are damaged (e.g., by UV radiation, trauma, inflammation) the entire cell ensemble enters a state of excitation and begins to produce a huge number of mediators, the effect of which is almost impossible to trace. No model system can account for all the processes and signaling pathways in the skin. This is another strong argument in favor of soft effects that do not allow for traumatizing the skin or weakening its protective structures.

In addition, people with fair skin from birth should remember that even a tan does not protect skin cells from damage since the melanin of Caucasoid skin is not a very reliable UV filter and, in some cases, it can even be an "assistant" to aggressive UV light. For white people, the sun is an ever-present harmful factor that causes premature skin aging and melanoma development. Dark skin contains more active melanocytes, and melanin reliably protects cell DNA from UV radiation. But beauticians, when approached by clients with ethnic skin dreaming of looking like the Europeans, should be aware that by trying to whiten dark skin, they engage in combat with a powerful anti-stress system that has been hardened in battle and is always ready to fight against any unwelcome intervention. Any local procedures in these people can lead to post-inflammatory hyperpigmentation.

As was shown in this book, to develop an effective and safe program of pigmentation treatment, it is essential to consider the following factors:

- Accurate diagnosis
- Understanding the skin physiology and melanogenesis
- Well-chosen combined step-by-step approach — reducing the background activity of melanocytes, destruction of existing pigment and inhibition of new pigment formation, acceleration of melanin elimination with exfoliating methods, skin protection
- Careful observance of all recommendations for the patient's home skincare
- Readiness for long-term treatment

You will find all the basic information in our book. All that's left to do is to implement what you've learned in the fight against pigmentation lesions.

References

Achar A., Rathi S.K. Melasma: a clinico-epidemiological study of 312 cases. Indian J Dermatol 2011; 569(4): 380–382.

Alaluf S., Atkins D., Barrett K. et al. Ethnic variation in melanin content and composition in photoexposed and photoprotected human skin. Pigment Cell Res 2002; 15(2): 112–118.

Alaluf S., Barrett K., Blount M., Carter N. Ethnic variation in tyrosinase and TYRP1 expression in photoexposed and photoprotected human skin. Pigment Cell Res 2003; 16(1): 35–42.

Al Ghamdi K.M., Kumar A., Al-Rikabi A.C., Mubarak M. Safety and efficacy of parenteral glutathione as a promising skin lightening agent: a controlled assessor-blinded pharmacohistologic and ultrastructural study in an animal model. Dermatol Ther 2020; 33(2): e13211.

Arjinpathana N., Asawanonda P. Glutathione as an oral whitening agent: a randomized, double-blind, placebo-controlled study. J Dermatolog Treat 2012; 23(2): 97–102.

Balak D.M.W. Topical trifarotene: a new retinoid. Br J Dermatol 2018; 179(2): 231–232.

Baldea I., Mocan T., Cosgarea R. The role of ultraviolet radiation and tyrosine stimulated melanogenesis in the induction of oxidative stress alterations in fair skin melanocytes. Exp Oncol 2009; 31(4): 200–208.

Balina L.M., Graupe K. The treatment of melasma. 20% azelaic acid versus 4% hydroquinone cream. Int J Dermatol 1991; 30(12): 893–895.

Bauer J., Bahmer F.A., Worl J. et al. A strikingly constant ratio exists between Langerhans cells and other epidermal cells in human skin: a stereologic study using the optical disector method and the confocal laser scanning microscope. J Invest Dermatol 2001; 116(2): 313–318.

Bauer J., Weng J., Kebebew E. et al. Germline variation of the melanocortin-1 receptor does not explain shared risk for melanoma and thyroid cancer. Exp Dermatol 2009; 18(6): 548–552.

Becatti M., Fiorillo C., Barygina V. et al. SIRT1 regulates MAPK pathways in vitiligo skin: insight into the molecular pathways of cell survival. J Cell Mol Med 2014; 18(3): 514–529.

Belote R.L., Simon S.M. Ca2+ transients in melanocyte dendrites and dendritic spine-like structures evoked by cell-to-cell signaling. J Cell Biol 2020; 219(1): e201902014.

Bento-Lopes L., Cabaço L.C., Charneca J., et al. Melanin's journey from melano-cytes to keratinocytes: uncovering the molecular mechanisms of melanin transfer and processing. Int J Mol Sci 2023; 24(14): 11289.

Bismuth K., Debbache J., Sommer L., Arnheiter H. Neural crest cell diversification and specification: melanocytes. Reference Module in Neuroscience and Biobe-havioral Psychology. Elsevier, 2017.

Boissy R.E., Visscher M., DeLong M.A. Deoxyarbutin: a novel reversible tyrosinase inhibitor with effective in vivo skin lightening potency. Exp Dermatol 2005; 14(8): 601–608.

Budamakuntla L., Loganathan E., Suresh D.H. et al. A randomised, open-label, comparative study of tranexamic acid microinjections and tranexamic acid with microneedling in patients with melasma. J Cutan Aesthet Surg 2013; 6(3): 139–143.

Bustamante J., Bredeston L., Malanga G., Mordoh J. Role of melanin as a scavenger of active oxygen species. Pigment Cell Res 1993; 6(5): 348–353.

Cayırlı M., Calışkan E., Açıkgöz G. et al. Regression of melasma with platelet-rich plasma treatment. Ann Dermatol 2014; 26(3): 401–402.

Cestari T.F., Dantas L.P., Boza J.C. Acquired hyperpigmentations. An Bras Dermatol 2014; 89(1): 11–25.

Charalambides M., Kibbi N., Young A.R. Effect of sunscreen application under max-imal-use conditions on plasma concentration of sunscreen active ingredients: a critical appraisal. Br J Dermatol 2020; 182(6): 1345–1347.

Chhabra G., Garvey D.R., Singh C.K. et al. Effects and mechanism of nicotinamide against UVA- and/or UVB-mediated DNA damage in normal melanocytes. Photochem Photobiol 2019; 95(1): 331–337.

Cho Y.H., Park J.E., Lim D.S., Lee J.S. Tranexamic acid inhibits melanogenesis by activating the autophagy system in cultured melanoma cells. J Dermatol Sci 2017; 88(1): 96–102.

Choudhry S.Z., Bhatia N., Ceilley R. et al. Role of oral Polypodium leucotomos ex-tract in dermatologic diseases: a review of the literature. J Drugs Dermatol 2014; 13(2): 148–153.

Cichorek M., Wachulska M., Stasiewicz A., Tymińska A. Skin melanocytes: biology and development. Postepy Dermatol Alergol 2013; 30(1): 30–41.

Damian D.L., Barnetson R.S., Halliday G.M. Measurement of in vivo sunscreen im-mune protection factors in humans. Photochem Photobiol 1999; 70(6): 910–915.

Dantas L.P., Boza J.C. Acquired hyperpigmentations. An Bras Dermatol 2014; 89(1): 11–25.

Davis E.C., Callender V.D. Post-inflammatory hyperpigmentation: a review of the epidemiology, clinical features, and treatment options in skin of color. J Clin Aesthet Dermatol 2010; 3(7): 20–31.

Del Bino S., Bernerd F. Variations in skin colour and the biological consequences of ultraviolet radiation exposure. Br J Dermatol 2013; 169(Suppl 3): 33–40.

Del Bino S., Duval C., Bernerd F. Clinical and biological characterization of skin pigmentation diversity and its consequences on UV impact. Int J Mol Sci 2018; 19(9): 2668.

Delinasios G.J., Karbaschi M., Cooke M.S., Young A.R. Vitamin E inhibits the UVAI induction of "light" and "dark" cyclobutane pyrimidine dimers, and oxidatively generated DNA damage, in keratinocytes. Sci Rep 2018; 8(1): 423.

Del Rosso J.Q. Polypodium Leucotomos Extract (PLE): New study gives evidence-based insight into "Ain't nothing like the real thing." J Clin Aesthet Dermatol 2019; 12(8): 45–46.

Deri B., Kanteev M., Goldfeder M. et al. The unravelling of the complex pattern of tyrosinase inhibition. Sci Rep 2016; 6: 34993.

Dina Y., McKesey J., Pandya A.G. Disorders of hypopigmentation. J Drugs Dermatol 2019; 18(3): 115–116.

D'Orazio J., Jarrett S., Amaro-Ortiz A., Scott T. UV radiation and the skin. Int J Mol Sci 2013; 14(6): 12222–12248.

Duteil L., Cardot-Leccia N., Queille-Roussel C. et al. Differences in visible light-induced pigmentation according to wavelengths: a clinical and histological study in comparison with UVB exposure. Pigment Cell Melanoma Res 2014; 27(5): 822–826.

Duteil L., Esdaile J., Maubert Y. et al. A method to assess the protective efficacy of sunscreens against visible light-induced pigmentation. Photodermatol Photoimmunol Photomed 2017; 33(5): 260–266.

Ebanks J.P., Wickett R.R., Boissy R.E. Mechanisms regulating skin pigmentation: the rise and fall of complexion coloration. Int J Mol Sci 2009; 10(9): 4066–4087.

Elias P.M. Stratum corneum defensive functions: an integrated view. J Invest Dermatol 2005; 125(2): 183–200.

Esmat S.M., El-Tawdy A.M., Hafez G.A. et al. Acral lesions of vitiligo: why are they resistant to photochemotherapy? J Eur Acad Dermatol Venereol 2012; 26(9): 1097–1104.

Finamor D.C., Sinigaglia-Coimbra R, Neves L.C. et al. A pilot study assessing the effect of prolonged administration of high daily doses of vitamin D on the clinical course of vitiligo and psoriasis. Dermatoendocrinol 2013; 5(1): 222–234.

Forbat E., Al-Niaimi F., Ali F.R. Use of nicotinamide in dermatology. Clin Exp Dermatol 2017; 42(2): 137–144.

George A. Tranexamic acid: an emerging depigmenting agent Pigment Int 2016; 3(2): 66–71.

Goh C.-L., Chuah S.Y., Tien S. et al. Double-blind, placebo-controlled trial to evaluate the effectiveness of Polypodium leucotomos extract in the treatment of melasma in Asian skin. A pilot study. J Clin Aesthet Dermatol 2018; 11(3): 14–19.

Goldman L., Igelman J., Richfield D. Impact of the laser on nevi and melanomas. Arch Dermatol 1964; 90: 71–75.

Goldstein N.B., Koster M.I., Hoaglin L.G. et al. Narrow band ultraviolet B treatment for human vitiligo is associated with proliferation, migration, and differentiation of melanocyte precursors. J Invest Dermatol 2015; 135(8): 2068–2076.

Hanada Y., Berbari E.F., Steckelberg J.M. Minocycline-induced cutaneous hyperpigmentation in an orthopedic patient population. Open Forum Infect Dis 2016; 3(1): ofv107.

Hasegawa K., Fujiwara R., Sato K. et al. Possible involvement of keratinocyte growth factor in the persistence of hyperpigmentation in both human facial solar lentigines and melasma. Ann Dermatol 2015; 27(5): 626–629.

Hollick E.J., Igwe C., Papamichael E. et al. Corneal and scleral problems caused by skin-lightening creams. Cornea 2019; 38(10): 1332–1335.

Hou A., Cohen B., Haimovic A., Elbuluk N. Microneedling: a comprehensive review. Dermatol Surg 2017; 43(3): 321–339.

Hüls A., Vierkötter A., Gao W. et al. Traffic-related air pollution contributes to development of facial lentigines: further epidemiological evidence from Caucasians and Asians. J Invest Dermatol 2016; 136(5): 1053–1056.

Hurbain I., Romao M., Sextius P. et al. Melanosome distribution in keratinocytes in different skin types: melanosome clusters are not degradative organelles. J Invest Dermatol 2018; 138(3): 647–656.

Ismail E.S.A., Patsatsi A., Abd El-Maged W.M., Nada E.E.A.E. Efficacy of microneedling with topical vitamin C in the treatment of melasma. J Cosmet Dermatol 2019; 18(5): 1342–1347.

Jablonski N.G., Chaplin G. Colloquium paper: human skin pigmentation as an adaptation to UV radiation. Proc Natl Acad Sci USA 2010a; 107(Suppl 2): 8962–8968.

Jablonski N.G., Chaplin G. In the light of evolution. Volume IV: The Human Condition. Edited by Avise J.C. and Ayala F.J. Washington National Academies Press, 2010b.

Janney M.S., Subramaniyan R., Dabas R. et al. A randomized controlled study comparing the efficacy of topical 5% tranexamic acid solution versus 3% hydroquinone cream in melasma. J Cutan Aesthet Surg 2019; 12(1): 63–67.

Jee S.H., Lee S.Y., Chiu H.C. et al. Effects of estrogen and estrogen receptor in normal human melanocytes. Biochem Biophys Res Commun 1994; 199: 1407–1412.

Juhasz M.L.W., Levin M.K. The role of systemic treatments for skin lightening. J Cosmet Dermatol 2018; 17(6): 1144–1157.

Kadekaro A.L., Wakamatsu K., Ito S., Abdel-Malek Z.A. Cutaneous photoprotection and melanoma susceptibility: reaching beyond melanin content to the frontiers of DNA repair. Front Biosci 2006; 11: 2157–2173.

Kaidbey K.H., Agin P.P., Sayre R.M., Kligman A.M. Photoprotection by melanin — a comparison of black and Caucasian skin. J Am Acad Dermatol 1979; 1: 249–260.

Kaya G., Tran C., Sorg O. et al. Hyaluronate fragments reverse skin atrophy by a CD44-dependent mechanism. PLoS Med 2006; 3(12): e493.

Kim M.S., Bang S.H., Kim J.H. et al. Tranexamic acid diminishes laser-induced melanogenesis. Ann Dermatol 2015; 27(3): 250–256.

Kim S.J., Park J.Y., Shibata T. et al. Efficacy and possible mechanisms of topical tranexamic acid in melasma. Clin Exp Dermatol 2016; 41(5): 480–485.

Krutmann J., Passeron T., Gilaberte Y. et al. Photoprotection of the future: challenges and opportunities. J Eur Acad Dermatol Venereol 2020; 34(3): 447–454.

Kuehn B. Mercury poisoning from skin cream. JAMA 2020; 323(6): 500.

Lan C.C., Wu C.S., Chiou M.H. et al. Low-energy helium-neon laser induces melanocyte proliferation via interaction with type IV collagen: visible light as a therapeutic option for vitiligo. Br J Dermatol 2009; 161(2): 273–280.

Lancer H.A. Lancer Ethnicity Scale (LES). Lasers Surg Med 1998; 22(1): 9.

Lee H.C., Thng T.G., Goh C.L. Oral tranexamic acid (TA) in the treatment of melasma: a retrospective analysis. J Am Acad Dermatol 2016; 75(2): 385–392.

Lin T.K., Zhong L., Santiago J.L. Association between stress and the HPA axis in the atopic dermatitis. Int J Mol Sci 2017; 18(10): 2131.

Lourenco E.A.J., Shaw L., Pratt H. et al. Application of SPF moisturisers is inferior to sunscreens in coverage of facial and eyelid regions. PLoS One 2019; 14(4): e0212548.

Lucock M.D. The evolution of human skin pigmentation: a changing medley of vitamins, genetic variability, and UV radiation during human expansion. Am J Biol Anthropol 2022; 180(2): 252–271.

Maeda K., Hatao M. Involvement of photooxidation of melanogenic precursors in prolonged pigmentation induced by ultraviolet A. J Invest Dermatol 2004; 122(2): 503–509.

Mahmoud B.H., Ruvolo E., Hexsel C.L. et al. Impact of long-wavelength UVA and visible light on melanocompetent skin. J Invest Dermatol 2010; 130(8): 2092–2097.

Makino E.T., Mehta R.C., Banga A. et al. Evaluation of a hydroquinone-free skin brightening product using in vitro inhibition of melanogenesis and clinical reduction of ultraviolet-induced hyperpigmentation. J Drugs Dermatol 2013; 12(3): S16–S20.

Matta M.K., Florian J., Zusterzeel R. et al. Effect of sunscreen application on plasma concentration of sunscreen active ingredients: a randomized clinical trial. JAMA 2020; 323(3): 256–267.

Matta M.K., Zusterzeel R., Pilli N.R. et al. Effect of sunscreen application under maximal use conditions on plasma concentration of sunscreen active ingredients: a randomized clinical trial. JAMA 2019; 321(21): 2082–2091.

McGregor D. Hydroquinone: an evaluation of the human risks from its carcinogenic and mutagenic properties. Crit Rev Toxicol 2007; 37(10): 887–914.

Mei X.L., Wang L. Ablative fractional carbon dioxide laser combined with intense pulsed light for the treatment of photoaging skin in Chinese population: a split-face study. Medicine (Baltimore) 2018; 97(3): e9494.

Menon A., Eram H., Kamath P.R. et al. A split-face comparative study of safety and efficacy of microneedling with tranexamic acid versus microneedling with vitamin C in the treatment of melasma. Indian Dermatol Online J 2019; 11(1): 41–45.

Middelkamp-Hup M.A., Pathak M.A., Parrado C. et al. Orally administered Polypodium leucotomos extract decreases psoralen–UVA-induced phototoxicity, pigmentation, and damage of human skin. J Am Acad Dermatol 2004; 50(1): 41–49.

Miri A., Akbarpour Birjandi S., Sarani M. Survey of cytotoxic and UV protection effects of biosynthesized cerium oxide nanoparticles. J Biochem Mol Toxicol 2020; 34(6): e22475.

Mohiuddin A.K. Skin lightening & management of hyperpigmentation. Pharm Sci Analytical Res J 2019; 2(2): 180020.

Na J.I., Shin J.W., Choi H.R. et al. Resveratrol as a multifunctional topical hypopigmenting agent. Int J Mol Sci 2019; 20(4): 956.

Nestor M., Bucay V., Callender V. et al. Polypodium leucotomos as an adjunct treatment of pigmentary disorders. J Clin Aesthet Dermatol 2014; 7(3): 13–17.

Nordlund J.J. The melanocyte and the epidermal melanin unit: an expanded concept. Dermatol Clin 2007; 25(3): 271–281.

Ozdeslik R.N., Olinski L.E., Trieu M.M. et al. Human nonvisual opsin 3 regulates pigmentation of epidermal melanocytes through functional interaction with melanocortin 1 receptor. Proc Natl Acad Sci USA 2019; 116(23): 11508–11517.

Panzella L., Ebato A., Napolitano A., Koike K. The late stages of melanogenesis: exploring the chemical facets and the application opportunities. Int J Mol Sci 2018; 19(6): 1753.

Panzella L., Leone L., Greco G. et al. Red human hair pheomelanin is a potent pro-oxidant mediating UV-independent contributory mechanisms of melanoma-genesis. Pigment Cell Melanoma Res 2014; 27(2): 244–252.

Park H.J., Cho J.H., Hong S.H. et al. Whitening and anti-wrinkle activities of ferulic acid isolated from Tetragonia tetragonioides in B16F10 melanoma and CCD-986sk fibroblast cells. J Nat Med 2018; 72(1): 127–135.

Parrado C., Mascaraque M., Gilaberte Y. et al. Fernblock (Polypodium leucotomos extract): molecular mechanisms and pleiotropic effects in light-related skin conditions. Photoaging and skin cancers, a review. Int J Mol Sci 2016; 17(7): 1026.

Parrado C., Mercado-Saenz S., Perez-Davo A. et al. Environmental stressors on skin aging. Mechanistic insights. Front Pharmacol 2019; 10: 759.

Parvez S., Kang M., Chung H.S. et al. Survey and mechanism of skin depigmenting and lightening agents. Phytother Res 2006; 20(11): 921–934.

Pathak M.A., Riley F.C., Fitzpatrick T.B. Melanogenesis in human skin following exposure to long-wave ultraviolet and visible light. J Invest Dermatol 1962a; 39: 435–443.

Pathak M.A., Riley F.J., Fitzpatrick T.B., Curwen W.L. Melanin formation in human skin induced by long-wave ultra-violet and visible light. Nature 1962b; 193: 148–150.

Pellosi M.C., Suzukawa A.A., Scalfo A.C., et al. Effects of the melanin precursor 5,6-dihydroxy-indole-2-carboxylic acid (DHICA) on DNA damage and repair in the presence of reactive oxygen species. Arch Biochem Biophys 2014; 557: 55–64.

Peng F., Tsuji G., Zhang J.Z. et al. Potential role of PM2.5 in melanogenesis. Environ Int 2019; 132: 105063.

Penney K.B., Smith C.J., Allen J.C. Depigmenting action of hydroquinone depends on disruption of fundamental cell processes. J Invest Dermatol 1984; 82(4): 308–310.

Peres D.D., Sarruf F.D., de Oliveira C.A. et al. Ferulic acid photoprotective properties in association with UV filters: multifunctional sunscreen with improved SPF and UVA-PF. J Photochem Photobiol B 2018; 185: 46–49.

Pillaiyar T., Namasivayam. V, Manickam M., Jung S.H. Inhibitors of melanogenesis: an updated review. J Med Chem 2018; 61(17): 7395–7418.

Piña-Oviedo S., Ortiz-Hidalgo C., Ayala A.G. Human colors – The rainbow garden of pathology: what gives normal and pathologic tissues their color? Arch Pathol Lab Med 2017; 141(3): 445–462.

Ramaut L., Hoeksema H., Pirayesh A. et al. Microneedling: where do we stand now? A systematic review of the literature. J Plast Reconstr Aesthet Surg 2018; 71(1): 1–14.

Raposo G., Marks M.S. The dark side of lysosome-related organelles: specialization of the endocytic pathway for melanosome biogenesis. Traffic 2002; 3(4): 237–248.

Raulin C., Karsai S. Laser and IPL technology in dermatology and aesthetic medicine. Springer-Verlag Berlin Heidelberg 2011.

Regazzetti C., Sormani L., Debayle D. et al. Melanocytes sense blue light and regulate pigmentation through opsin-3. J Invest Dermatol 2018; 138(1): 171–178.

Sánchez-Pérez J.F., Vicente-Agullo D., Barberá M. et al. Relationship between ultraviolet index (UVI) and first-, second- and third-degree sunburn using the Probit methodology. Sci Rep 2019; 9(1): 733.

Sarma N., Chakraborty S., Poojary S.A. et al. Evidence-based review, grade of recommendation, and suggested treatment recommendations for melasma. Indian Dermatol Online J 2017; 8(6): 406–442.

SCCS, Degen G.H. Opinion of the Scientific Committee on Consumer safety (SCCS) — Opinion on the safety of the use of deoxyarbutin in cosmetic products. Regul Toxicol Pharmacol 2016; 74: 77–78.

Serre C., Busuttil V., Botto J.M. Intrinsic and extrinsic regulation of human skin melanogenesis and pigmentation. Int J Cosmet Sci 2018; 40(4): 328–347.

Shah S., Chew S.K. Efficacy and safety of topical depigmenting agent in healthy human fair skin female volunteers: a single-arm study. J Cosmet Dermatol 2018; 17(5): 830–839.

Sirithanabadeekul P., Dannarongchai A., Suwanchinda A. Platelet-rich plasma treatment for melasma: a pilot study. J Cosmet Dermatol 2020; 19(6): 1321–1327.

Smit N.P., van Nieuwpoort F.A., Marrot L. et al. Increased melanogenesis is a risk factor for oxidative DNA damage — Study on cultured melanocytes and atypical nevus cells. Photochem Photobiol 2008; 84(3): 550–555.

Solano F. Melanins: skin pigments and much more — types, structural models, biological functions, and formation routes. New J Sci 2014; Article ID 498276.

Sondenheimer K., Krutmann J. Novel means for photoprotection. Front Med (Lausanne) 2018; 5: 162.

Sparavigna A., Tenconi B., De Ponti I. Antiaging, photoprotective, and brightening activity in biorevitalization: a new solution for aging skin. Clin Cosmet Investig Dermatol 2015; 8: 57–65.

Swope V.B., Abdel-Malek Z.A. MC1R: front and center in the bright side of dark eumelanin and DNA repair. Int J Mol Sci 2018; 19(9): 2667.

Talagas M., Misery L. Role of keratinocytes in sensitive skin. Front Med (Lausanne) 2019; 6: 108.

Taylor S., Grimes P., Lim J. et al. Postinflammatory hyperpigmentation. J Cutan Med Surg 2009; 13(4): 183–191.

Thingnes J., Lavelle T.J., Hovig E., Omholt S.W. Understanding the melanocyte distribution in human epidermis: an agent-based computational model approach. PLoS One 2012; 7(7): e40377.

Tobin D.J. The cell biology of human hair follicle pigmentation. Pigment Cell Melanoma Res 2011; 24(1): 75–88.

Tomita Y., Maeda K., Tagami H. Melanocyte-stimulating properties of arachidonic acid metabolites: possible role in postinflammatory pigmentation. Pigment Cell Res 1992; 5(5 Pt 2): 357–361.

Uysal C.A., Ertas N.M. Platelet-rich plasma increases pigmentation. J Craniofac Surg 2017; 28(8): e793.

Valverde P., Healy E., Jackson I. et al. Variants of the melanocyte-stimulating hormone receptor gene are associated with red hair and fair skin in humans. Nat Genet 1995; 11(3): 328–330.

van Praag M.C., Roza L., Boom B.W. et al. Determination of the photoprotective efficacy of a topical sunscreen against UVB-induced DNA damage in human epidermis. J Photochem Photobiol B 1993; 19(2): 129–134.

Victorelli S., Lagnado A., Halim J. et al. Senescent human melanocytes drive skin ageing via paracrine telomere dysfunction. EMBO J 2019; 38(23): 101982.

Vierkötter A., Schikowski T., Ranft U. et al. Airborne particle exposure and extrinsic skin aging. J Invest Dermatol 2010;130(12): 2719–2726.

Visscher M.O. Skin color and pigmentation in ethnic skin. Facial Plast Surg Clin North Am 2017; 25(1): 119–125.

Weschawalit S., Thongthip S., Phutrakool P., Asawanonda P. Glutathione and its antiaging and antimelanogenic effects. Clin Cosmet Investig Dermatol 2017; 10: 147–153.

Wiel C., Le Gal K., Ibrahim M.X. et al. Stabilization by antioxidants stimulates lung cancer metastasis. Cell 2019; 178(2): 330–345.

Wolf Horrell E.M., Boulanger M.C., D'Orazio J.A. Melanocortin 1 receptor: structure, function, and regulation. Front Genet 2016; 7: 95.

Yuan X.H., Jin Z.H. Paracrine regulation of melanogenesis. Br J Dermatol 2018; 178(3): 632–639.

Zaidi K.U., Ali A.S., Ali S.A., Naaz I. Microbial tyrosinases: promising enzymes for pharmaceutical, food bioprocessing, and environmental industry. Biochem Res Int 2014; 2014: 854687.

Zhou H., Zhao J., Li A., Reetz M.T. Chemical and biocatalytic routes to arbutin. Molecules 2019; 24(18): 3303.

Zhou Y., Banga A.K. Enhanced delivery of cosmeceuticals by microdermabrasion. J Cosmet Dermatol 2011; 10(3): 179–184.

Zubair S., Mujtaba G. Comparison of efficacy of topical 2% liquiritin, topical 4% liquiritin and topical 4% hydroquinone in the management of melasma. J Pakistan Assoc Derm 2009; 19: 158–163.

www.ingramcontent.com/pod-product-compliance
Lightning Source LLC
Chambersburg PA
CBHW052019030426
42335CB00026B/3211